PROFILES IN MENTAL HEALTH COURAGE

Also by Patrick J. Kennedy & Stephen Fried

A Common Struggle

Also by Stephen Fried

Rush

Appetite for America

Thing of Beauty

The New Rabbi

Bitter Pills

Husbandry

PROFILES IN MENTAL HEALTH COURAGE

✳

PATRICK J. KENNEDY

& STEPHEN FRIED

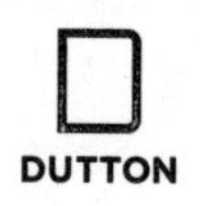

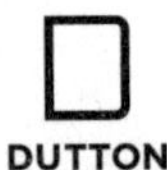

DUTTON
An imprint of Penguin Random House LLC
penguinrandomhouse.com

LIBRARY OF CONGRESS CATALOGING-IN-PUBLICATION DATA

Names: Kennedy, Patrick J. (Patrick Joseph), author. | Fried, Stephen, author.
Title: Profiles in mental health courage / Patrick J. Kennedy & Stephen Fried.
Description: [New York] : Dutton, [2024]
Identifiers: LCCN 2023058101 (print) | LCCN 2023058102 (ebook) | ISBN 9780593471760 (hardcover) | ISBN 9780593471784 (epub)
Subjects: LCSH: Mentally ill—United States—Biography. | Recovering addicts—United States—Biography. | Psychotherapy patients—United States—Biography. | Mental illness—United States—Popular works. | Mental health—United States—Popular works.
Classification: LCC RC464.A1 K46 2024 (print) | LCC RC464.A1 (ebook) | DDC 362.29092/2—dc23/eng/20240123
LC record available at https://lccn.loc.gov/2023058101
LC ebook record available at https://lccn.loc.gov/2023058102

Printed in the United States of America
1st Printing

To those still suffering in silence

Contents

CONTENTS

PROFILES IN MENTAL HEALTH COURAGE

Prologue

In 1956, my uncle John F. Kennedy, then a U.S. senator, wrote a book that is probably more famous for its great title than its contents. It was called *Profiles in Courage*. And it was about eight U.S. senators who JFK felt had made particularly courageous contributions to American history.

For a while now, I have been thinking about what courage means to me. While growing up with my father, Ted Kennedy, in the Senate, and then serving in the House of Representatives myself for many years, I saw quite a bit of bravery in politics. But the truth is, the most courageous people I know qualify not for what they do in public but what they are able to endure and rise above in private. This is especially true of people who struggle every day with mental illness, or addiction, or both, or who help loved ones or family members in their struggles.

The details and daily dramas of these struggles usually remain private, hidden. And even when people discuss them publicly, it's often in a brief or very cautious way—enough to admit to having a diagnosis or a problem, or "issues," in order to support advocacy, but rarely enough to inform a public that wants and *needs* to understand what living with these illnesses is like every day.

In 2015, I decided to share an in-depth narrative of my struggles with substance use disorders and mood disorders—along with the politics and discrimination that make these conditions harder to treat and live with than necessary.

This was not without risks. Several people extremely close to me warned that if I published the resulting book, *A Common Struggle,* my relationship with them would never be the same. Sadly, some of them did distance themselves from me—and I ache over those damaged or lost relationships. But for every person who all but closed me off from their life for being open, I met so many who did just the opposite. They led me to believe that sharing my truth had helped set them free with their own. Or, at the very least, that my complicated medical history had served to show people in their lives—siblings, spouses, bosses—that what they were going through was not so unique and, in fact, was shockingly common for people with these illnesses.

We often quote the statistic that, at any given time, at least a quarter of all Americans struggle with mental illness, substance use disorder, or both. And while these are still sometimes viewed as two separate illnesses—because two distinct worlds developed to address them—I can tell you as someone who has them both that they are best understood and treated together as one complex continuum of diseases of the brain and mind.

Unfortunately, the percentage of people affected by these illnesses is likely quite a bit higher than 25 percent. And the percentage of those who don't feel comfortable and supported enough to be open about their experiences is much, *much* higher, as is the percentage of those who cannot access or afford evidence-based care and support.

Each time a new statistic is released regarding the state of mental illness diagnoses, addictions to drug or alcohol, overdoses, suicide attempts, and completed suicides, it is followed by a call for a "new appreciation" of these illnesses, a "paradigm shift." But part of the paradigm we need to shift is the idea that these are new problems. If there is anything truly new about them, it is how much incrementally *worse* they have gotten because we have not done enough as a society to address them. Nor have we made sure that the treatments we already have, which aren't perfect but still can save lives, get delivered to most of the people who need them. Those treatments—which all work but have been proven to work best together—are medical therapies, talk therapies, and healing relationships (everything from recovery and support groups to faith groups). Even those getting some form of treatment might not be getting the most evidence-based or complete treatment, and there is often quite a difference between what is "approved" or "legal" and what is ideal.

This is an age-old problem. You only need to look at the historic figures JFK wrote about in *Profiles in Courage* to see it. At least half of them, going back to the earliest days of postrevolutionary America, were known to have struggled with mental illness or addiction, or had the struggle for mental wellness profoundly affect their families.

JOHN QUINCY ADAMS—WHOSE story first inspired JFK and his co-author, Ted Sorenson, to write *Profiles in Courage*—was nine years old when his father signed the Declaration of Independence, twenty-nine when his father became president, and thirty-five when he himself became a U.S. senator. John Quincy lost both of his younger brothers to alcoholism, beginning with Charles at age thirty. His father also suffered from depression, especially after the trauma of losing Charles and losing the presidential election to his friend Thomas Jefferson—all during the same week in late 1800. John Quincy's oldest son, George Washington Adams, suffered from depression and took his own life at the age of twenty-eight—just two months after his father's presidency ended in 1829. Not long after learning of his son's death, John Quincy vowed to use his "remaining days" for good works "tributary to the well-being of others" and soon became the first ex-president to rejoin the government as a congressman. But he continued to experience tragedy from mental illness. In 1832, his remaining brother, Thomas, died from complications of alcoholism at the age of fifty-nine. And two years after that, his own son John died from the same thing at the age of thirty-one.

Among the other seven JFK profiled, Massachusetts lawyer and politician Daniel Webster suffered from alcoholism and died from cirrhosis of the liver in 1852.

Sam Houston, a key figure in Texas independence—and the state's first president before becoming a senator—had a well-known battle with alcoholism and either depression or bipolar disorder. He may qualify as the nation's first case of political mental health stigma. His nickname among the Cherokee, with whom he had been close since childhood, was Oo-tse-tee Ar-dee-tah-skee, or "Big Drunk," and his drinking was an open, caustic issue in his public life. His third wife—who he married when she was twenty-one and he was forty-seven—made it her mission to help him remain sober, but his political adversaries continued to publicly shame him.

Lucius Lamar, the U.S. senator from Mississippi, was only nine years old when his namesake father, a prominent Georgia judge, took his own life, just days before his thirty-seventh birthday in 1834. He reportedly "entered his house, wrote a short farewell note to his family, and walked into the garden and shot himself in the head with his pistol."

And these are just the ones we know about and can begin to document.

None of this should be surprising. But somehow it still is. Our nation is experiencing perhaps its most pronounced crisis of mental illness and substance use disorders in history; already-high depression and anxiety rates rose another 25 percent worldwide after the first year of the COVID-19 pandemic. Yet, too many of us still don't understand what the experience of having or treating these diseases is like.

In our society, you don't have to have cancer, or heart disease, or diabetes, to understand the basic dynamics and challenges of living with these illnesses. Their treatment has become part of our culture, openly discussed and encouraged. But when it comes to diseases that affect the brain—cognition, mood, thought, impulsivity, self-destructiveness—we are surprised again and again, or ignorant in a way that isn't just unsupportive but can be downright dangerous.

AT THE HEIGHT of COVID, when Simone Biles announced she would not compete in the Summer Olympics to preserve her mental health, I was watching the public reaction with fascination and sadness. So was my *Common Struggle* co-author, award-winning medical journalist Stephen Fried, and we started texting about this. It seemed as if nobody wanted to know more about a health situation Biles had obviously been wrestling with for quite some time. All they wanted to know was why she couldn't perform the way they wanted her to—which is, of course, one of the biggest challenges of having these illnesses: people demanding to know why you just can't or just *won't* "snap out of it!"

A version of this takes place almost any time a public figure or a private person acknowledges a personal struggle with mental illness or addiction—often expressing a desire to take time away to treat it, or just asking for emotional support. There might be a moment of generic sympathy, a statement about how these illnesses aren't as stigmatized as they used to be (which some days I believe, and other days I'm not sure), but not much curiosity or care about their health treatment.

The inability of people to understand the actual challenges of these illnesses, and to learn about them and empathize with them, is as big an epidemic as the diseases themselves. Stephen and I decided we wanted to address this directly.

So we started talking about a book that would help empower those with mental illness and addiction, and help normalize their struggles, by finding untold stories all over the country and telling them in a more nuanced and honest way than is typical. We hoped that by doing so, we could help people see and appreciate these profiles in courage, even as those profiled continued to struggle.

We decided to find and feature more people than JFK had—courageous people with different mental illnesses and addictions from across the country. We sought diversity by age, race, gender, socioeconomic class, and diagnosis—even wellness.

We weren't looking for people to come out and offer an anecdote or two to support important advocacy causes. And we weren't looking for people who were telling a story primarily to endorse something—a medicine, a therapy, an app, a healer—that solved everything for them. (I am friends with many people who have done this, and I do respect them for taking the risk of coming out at all.)

Instead, we were looking for people who wanted to talk openly about doing well and not doing well, about the messy challenges—and even the messy successes—of living with these illnesses. Just as JFK had hoped to highlight "political courage" with his profiles, we wanted to honor and inspire all the different kinds of "mental health courage" it takes to keep going, keep trying, and keep starting over, seeking wellness and staying alive—along with the courage it takes to risk telling these stories in order to help America face its mental health crisis in our families, in our workplaces, in our jails, and on our streets.

And we also wanted to include those who had lost their courageous struggle, by taking their own lives, or accidentally overdosing.

We started reaching out to people in sports, media, politics, business, and medicine to find powerful untold stories of courage in the face of mental illness and addiction. We also reached out to caregivers, directors of mental health training and treatment programs, advocates, and their friends seeking recommendations and connections.

We reached out to my family members. There are some in treatment and many in recovery, and, sadly, we have lost two cousins, one to suicide and one to overdose, in just the past few years. We also reached out to some of the hundreds of people—some well-known, most not—who have, over the years, asked for my help.

I am awed by the people we have met through this journey. I am also awed by the people I already knew, but who never really spoke to me, or anyone else, in great depth about their challenges and courageous approaches to life. When they shared, I found myself sharing with them, about my own personal challenges with bipolar disorder and addiction.

I'm revealing this not because it's comfortable or comforting. It isn't. My wife, Amy, is sometimes apprehensive about my being this open. But she supports me because she knows this is how I cope with my illness and remain sober, for myself, for her, and for our kids. We are, as we're taught in our twelve-step meetings, "only as sick as our secrets." And if I'm asking others to "come out," the least I can do is try to meet them at each new level of honesty and self-revelation.

The level of openness, self-knowledge, and willingness to answer incredibly personal questions on the part of our profile subjects has, I must admit, continually blown me away. It has also very much reenergized me.

In the years after *A Common Struggle* was published in 2015, Amy and I had two more children—our fourth and fifth—and I dialed back some of my advocacy work in the face of a new administration that was fighting against the very expansion of medical care we had spent so long helping to create. I was asked to serve on a White House commission to combat opiate use, but when it became clear that no funding was being put toward the effort, I called the president out and then stepped down. I accepted more speaking engagements and some board positions for mental health innovators and made sure I could be home to help with the kids. Then, after our Democratic congressman switched parties, Amy decided to run for Congress herself in 2020, winning the Democratic primary and almost winning the election. When it was over, even though my friend Joe Biden was the new president, the country was in a pandemic, and we all went into quarantine. Starting this book a year later was a great reason to reconnect with so many people after the fog of COVID began to lift.

We talked to more than a hundred people, some multiple times, just to get ideas of possible profile subjects and different aspects of courage in the face of mental illness and addiction. I reached out to many people in my address book who I had previously worked with on these issues. (In one twenty-four-hour period, Stephen and I met with the heads of the National Institute of Mental Health, the

National Institute on Drug Abuse, and the National Institute on Alcohol Abuse and Alcoholism.)

We interviewed each profile subject many times. We also interviewed family members, caregivers, and friends, and in many situations we were able to review medical records and personal writing.

For the past two years, we have been keeping an enormous number of confidences. And we have never stopped being amazed at how people can sustain such high levels of function and dysfunction.

Some of the people in this book I have known for a long time but got to know much better through the interviews—talking about things I never even would have known, or dared, to ask about. Others we met through quiet networking, private recommendations, or complete coincidence. For each person you will meet on these pages, we spoke to many others. We promised anyone we interviewed that if they changed their minds about "coming out" this way at any point in the project, we would respect their wishes. Some did change their minds. And some had stories we felt were too complex or unresolved to present in this format. We thank them all for the time and energy they gave to this project and their belief in our goal of illuminating and normalizing the experience of struggling with mental health in this country.

Profiles in Mental Health Courage is meant to be read by people well-versed in the diagnosis and treatment of mental illness and addiction, as well as those who don't understand these worlds at all—because there is always hope that they might.

One of our profile subjects, a Nashville health-care aide in her thirties, told us about a recent conversation she had with her seventy-two-year-old father, who for decades has insisted her psychiatric symptoms were all "made up" and her multiple addictions were just "weakness." During what was probably her fiftieth lifetime hospitalization for psychiatric or substance use emergencies—and the third one during the time we had been interviewing her—she said her dad came to visit her during a detox at Vanderbilt University Hospital. And as they sat in low chairs in the family visiting room, she was stunned as he turned to her and said, "I'm startin' to think this thing is a *disease* that you have . . ."

This book is not meant to, in any way, judge anyone's choices or their learning curves. It is meant to show, in great factual and emotional depth, just how challenging these illnesses are. And, in many cases, the people who agreed to be profiled learned more about their own "lived experience" by being asked questions no one had ever asked them before and by exploring documentation they had never seen before.

One of our goals in writing this book was to make many aspects of dealing with these illnesses more understandable. And, by doing so, we hope to make people understand how much courage it takes to endure the daily struggles for continued or improved mental health.

Because, trust me, it takes courage. . . .

To admit to yourself you have a problem

To admit to a doctor or caregiver you have a problem

To admit to family and friends you have a problem

To find a treatment professional who you trust to help you

To pay for that professional

To get an initial diagnosis—realizing that because we still don't have the kind of diagnostic tests for mental health that we do for other diseases, the diagnosis is likely to be the starting point in a journey

To try a treatment that might work—whether you start with outpatient talk therapy or medication or support/recovery groups, or, if necessary, in more acute illness, inpatient care to protect from self-harm, detox from drugs or alcohol, or do more intensive diagnostic work

To deal with setbacks in treatment—worsening or changing of symptoms, adverse reactions to medication, relapses in recovery, changes in diagnosis

To deal with the impatience or lack of understanding of family, friends, and colleagues that you're having setbacks and your problem can't just be "cured"

To deal with your own impatience, anger, or sadness that you're having setbacks and your illness can't just be "cured"

To deal with the opportunities and life experiences deferred, lost, or ruined because of your illness

To deal with regrets

To deal with all the mixed media messages about mental health, and make personal decisions based on medical evidence and not politics or social commentaries (you can think too many people take antidepressants and still need an antidepressant yourself; you can think drug companies make too much money and still support treatments that can help stop people from taking their own lives)

To love and support those in our lives struggling with these illnesses, to forgive them when their struggles and setbacks make our lives more challenging, and to apologize to them when we realize we have been insensitive to their problems

To live in the face of statistics and systems that are stacked against you and your wellness.

HERE IS WHAT people with mental illness and substance use disorders, their families, their caregivers, and the health-care system are up against. Among American adults age eighteen and older:

One in four (84 million) had one or more mental disorders; one in twelve (28 million) had two or more mental disorders

One in ten (34 million) had one or more substance use disorders; one in fifty (6 million) had two or more substance use disorders

11 million had at least one mental disorder and at least one co-occurring substance use disorder

31.4 million had major depressive disorder

20.2 million had generalized anxiety disorder

3.7 million had a lifetime history of schizophrenia spectrum disorders (including schizophrenia, schizoaffective disorder, and schizophreniform disorder, also called "psychotic disorders," in which the dominant symptoms are delusions and hallucinations, as well as disorganized thinking, speech, and behavior)

2.5 million met diagnostic criteria for schizophrenia spectrum disorders in the past year (these schizophrenia spectrum numbers are more than twice as high as any previous estimate)

13.4 million met diagnostic criteria for alcohol use disorder in the past year

7.7 million had cannabis use disorder

3.2 million had a stimulant use disorder

1 million had an opioid use disorder

Only 60.8 percent of those with any mental disorder received treatment in the past year

Only 12.2 percent of those with any substance use disorder received treatment in the past year

This is the very latest data from the Department of Health and Human Services' new Mental and Substance Use Disorders Prevalence Study (MSDP) from 2022. This study is the first-ever attempt to gather incidence and treatment data with equal focus on mental illness and substance use disorders. It is also the first attempt to make sure that all Americans are represented in this data, including people who are incarcerated or experiencing homelessness.

These new numbers are vitally important. They can and should change some of our ideas about the incidence, severity, and impact of different mental illnesses and substance use disorders, including the prevention of premature deaths caused by them. But their equally important message, which is one we have tried to explore in telling these stories of mental health courage, is the amazing interconnectedness of these illnesses and their symptoms, and the endless challenge of diagnosing and treating these diseases as we are still learning so much about them.

WE WENT OUT of our way in this book to avoid being too analytical or wonky, resisting my endless desire to dig deeper and deeper into the policy mechanics and legal battles of assuring your right to health insurance parity for all mental illness and substance use disorder treatments. These rights were established by the Mental Health Parity and Addiction Equity Act of 2008, the bill I co-sponsored in the House and my father shepherded through the Senate not long before his death, and fortified by the Patient Protection and Affordable Care Act of 2010.

These protections include where you get your treatment: "inpatient" (in a hospital), "residential" (at a facility where you live during treatment), "outpatient" (where you visit a doctor's office or do telemedicine), and "partial hospitalization programs" or "intensive outpatient programs" (PHPs and IOPs, where you get individual and group therapy and other treatments at a facility for several hours a day, but sleep at home). They also include which treatments you receive: various forms of "talk therapy" (also called psychotherapy); psychoactive medicines, including medication-assisted treatment for addiction, being used on-label (for the diagnoses they're approved for), off-label, or experimentally, orally, by injection or infusion; procedures such as electroconvulsive therapy (ECT) and brain stimulation therapy; basically, whatever evidence-based treatment you and your mental health provider choose. (All medications in the book are listed by generic name first, then the relevant brand name.)

Our objective for this book was to tell stories of real people navigating the system, as well as their lives. We wanted only to explain what was needed to inform the storytelling. And whenever I started policy backsliding during the interviews, Stephen would remind me that we had already agreed to put a QR code and URL at the end of the book. They're on page 321, and can immediately connect readers to the Alignment for Progress site, where they'll find The Kennedy Forum's national strategy for mental health and substance disorders.

Reading these stories—unvarnished, powerful, sometimes inspiring, sometimes heartbreaking, often both—is a way of putting these trends and stats into perspective. When I first got into politics, and then got interested in mental health and substance use, I used a technique I had watched my father employ so successfully—local hearings, all over the country, where people could just tell their stories. During those hearings, I always wondered what it would be like to dig deeper into the most intriguing stories and include not just the raw "lived experience" of the person testifying but insights from other people around them, even the people they said were part of the problem. *Profiles in Mental Health Courage* has been an opportunity to do just that.

It is one of the great honors of my life that these twelve people trusted us to share their stories, daring to be truthful for no other reason than the hope that their frankness might help melt away some of the iciness of stigma and misunderstanding. We believe these profiles represent a new frontier in how we talk and think about mental health.

If you or someone you care about is experiencing a mental health emergency, call or text 988 for the national Suicide & Crisis Lifeline, or go online to chat at 988lifeline.org.

Chapter One

Philomena

Philomena Kebec is a crusading tribal rights, human rights, and public health attorney for the Bad River Band of the Lake Superior Tribe of Chippewa Indians. The forty-five-year-old lawyer lives in a small town just outside the reservation on the northern tip of Wisconsin with her daughter, her son, and her son's father. But she grew up in a bigger city in nearby Minneapolis, Minnesota—and her advocacy and fierce legal acumen are internationally known.

She has done everything from arguing as a staff attorney at the Indian Law Resource Center in Washington for the UN declaration of rights for all Indigenous peoples in the world to creating an innovative, hyperlocal, all-volunteer harm reduction and needle exchange program serving tribal and nontribal communities in northern Wisconsin.

One podcaster nicknamed her "the bad-ass woman from Bad River."

I was introduced to Philomena by my friend Michael Botticelli, the former director of National Drug Control Policy for the Obama administration and an addiction medicine expert who is in long-term recovery himself. He told me I should meet her, but he didn't want to say why.

Within minutes of talking to her, we had moved past her work, and she started discussing what had really been going on in her life. I immediately recognized that while she had been keeping a lot of her experiences to herself in her professional life, she was actually quite accustomed to talking about them—but primarily in the safety of twelve-step recovery meetings. People who share in meetings quickly connect to one another, regardless of the differences in age or circumstance.

I have always gone to tiny, private twelve-step meetings, first in D.C., with fellow public officials who couldn't be open enough about their addictions to risk being seen by the larger recovery public at a meeting.

(Throughout the book, I'm using "twelve-step" to refer to all types of regular peer support meetings for addictions. These originated in the 1930s when "Bill W." wrote out the twelve steps and created Alcoholics Anonymous, later followed by Narcotics Anonymous and groups for loved ones. There are now many twelve-step groups not affiliated with AA or NA, or strictly following their traditional insistence on secrecy and discouragement of psychiatric and addiction medications. So I'm using the general term.)

Philomena told me she had been in recovery since the age of seventeen, when she stopped binge drinking and smoking pot to such extremes that she once even stole her grandmother's sacred ceremonial pipe and used it to get high. But after college, when she was working in a bookstore and trying to figure out what to do with her life, she started attending a very large, long-standing meeting in Minneapolis called the Central Pacific. On Thursdays, that meeting would often attract three hundred people and be recorded. So sharing there was a uniquely private yet very public experience.

That big Central Pacific meeting changed Philomena's life in many ways beyond just helping her maintain her sobriety. It was through the meeting that she met the lawyer who hired her as a paralegal, then helped her get into law school and mentored her as an attorney.

She also refined her advocacy voice at the podium of the Thursday Central Pacific meeting. And nobody who was there that night ever forgot the story she told about the very last time she was abused by her stepfather at the age of twelve—a sharing that I heard about from someone else who was there.

She spoke for more than a half hour with searing, contagious passion, somehow managing to keep to the house rule of "no profanity from the podium." And then she tried to sum up by describing how she made sense of her feelings about her abuser.

"I've prayed a lot," she said, "and I've talked in recovery a lot about how to respond to that . . . to that . . ."

She stopped, total silence, mouth to the microphone, looking out at the audience into people's eyes, for more than a minute. It took forever.

And then she said, "To that . . . *motherfucker*!"

The whole room just exploded. "*Yes*," people were yelling, "*yes!*"

But having that kind of effect on people can come at a price. And while Philomena has been solid in her recovery for over twenty-five years, those closest to her know that the rest of her mental health has continued to be challenging. Part of the reason she's such an effective legal advocate may be that her emotions are so close to the surface; on controversial issues, she doesn't let go when others might, because she *can't let go*.

"Even today," she told me, "I go through periods where I get really emotionally spun out, really overwhelmed, and I can't stop crying. I would get cycles of obsessive thoughts, just creating this emotional whirlwind. At this time last year, I was suicidal. I was struggling with a diagnosis of major depression and PTSD. But a lot of that was brought on by workplace stress, too.

"Sometimes the only really effective way of getting out of one of these tailspins has been to engage in suicidal ideation or to cut myself—as I have since I was a teenager. It just ends up taking the wind out of it. And I think what happens, and I've talked to my therapist about this, is when I'm planning my death, my frontal lobe gets engaged in something else, and I'm able to get some relief from the emotional turmoil that's happening in other parts of my brain. I believe this is connected to my PTSD. And it's really terrifying. The whole thing is really terrifying."

Because of the nature of her work doing human rights law, she can actually view what is happening to her through different prisms, different worldviews for approaching trauma, mental illness, and addiction.

She learned early on about the traditional twelve-step prism, which would view the main way to address her challenges as simply abstaining from substance use and working the steps. She also came to understand there was a more psychiatric model of treating symptoms and illnesses with talk therapy, which she likes, and medication, which she would prefer not to take but has. Later in her career as a local advocate for health care during the opiate crisis, she got interested in the controversial model of harm reduction and needle exchange—creating safe places for addicts to use opiates, with naloxone (Narcan) on hand to reverse overdoses, and offering sterile injection equipment to lessen the chance of infection. (The harm reduction world is also more open to people taking medication to get off drugs or replace them.) And then there's the more recent idea of using "brain differences" or "neurodivergence" to recast mental illnesses and substance use disorders so they are seen not as diseases or medical conditions but as part of a spectrum of brain functionality.

These different worldviews are crucially important in fighting for human rights—disability rights, health insurance rights, LGBTQ+ rights, tribal rights. But appreciating them all can make the process of understanding what's wrong with you, and how it should be treated, fairly confusing. Especially when you add the pressures of the outside world to the pressures of your interior world.

"Here's how I see myself," she told me. "I'm an attorney who has been practicing for fifteen years. And I'm a person that has struggled with mental illness—and I still struggle with mental illness. Or, while I don't like that dichotomy, I do have mental differences."

She also brings the unique perspectives of tribal culture and medicine to the equation. It is not uncommon for people with mental health problems to wish for a more "natural" or "spiritual" way to address them. But they don't always know how to accomplish that: sometimes those who offer alternative help don't "believe" in traditional Western mental health medicine and expect people to choose between options that are, honestly, best used together. Psychiatric care and prayer, for example, are a great match: prayer *instead* of psychiatric care can be dangerous, even deadly.

Philomena was brought up in both Western and tribal cultures. At the moment, her treatment is being overseen by a psychiatric nurse practitioner on the reservation. These specially trained nurse practitioners (NPs)—also called psychiatric-mental health nurse practitioners—are licensed to write prescriptions (primarily for mental health care). But her nurse practitioner also expects that Philomena will seek out traditional Native ceremonies and treatments. These can include prayers, herbal medicines (swallowed, smoked, or smudged), sweat lodge sessions, or ceremonially "putting down tobacco" at the base of a tree—which is done when asking for assistance or permission.

"When I'm having a hard time, I'll go out and put some tobacco down and ask for pity," she explained. "I ask for love. I ask for direction."

Yet her nurse practitioner also expects that if Philomena needs talk therapy, she will get it. And if she needs a prescription medicine for her sleep disorders and her depression, she will take it.

"Mental illness can be a spiritual sickness," Philomena said, "but there are also Native words for *sadness* and *depression*."

GROWING UP, PHILOMENA, an only child, lived a fairly assimilated life with her mother; they moved from Chicago to Minneapolis when Philomena was three and her parents divorced. Her father was a prominent Chicago attorney who struggled with bipolar disorder and, later, kidney disease from longtime use of lithium. Her mother was a corporate communications specialist at Xcel Energy who struggled with alcohol use and later became a regular at Minneapolis area AA meetings. Philomena was close to her maternal grandmother, a teacher, and spent childhood summers with her at her home near the reservation, which was three hours away in northern Wisconsin, along Lake Superior.

She recalled her sexual abuse beginning at age eight or nine, when her stepfather, who took care of her in the afternoons because her mom was working full-time and also getting her MBA, created a new rule: she had to take a bath every day after school. When she tried to resist this, he hit her. "Much later," she told me, "I realized these beatings were to put the fear of God in me, to keep me from speaking about the abuse. I knew, at that young age, that he had a deadly level of rage. That he could lose it and kill me."

She recalled her mother initially being "oblivious" to what was happening, "buying into all of his stories and justifications" for hitting her, but she finally drew the line when "he lost his shit on me and beat me in front of the next-door neighbors." Since he blamed his behavior on drinking, the couple went into family outpatient treatment; Philomena, age eleven, and her mother participated as co-dependents in Al-Anon and Alateen. Not long after, her mother decided to join a twelve-step group for her own sobriety.

The situation finally came to a head during a family vacation in the Southwest. One night, her stepfather "started patting me on my chest," she remembered. "I was wearing one of my favorite T-shirts, from a Janet Jackson concert. I was irritated about that. We were supposed to go somewhere the next morning, and I didn't want to get up. When I finally did, he smacked the shit out of me—you know with certain people there's that emotional tornado that just happens very quickly. Once before, he had thrown me against a tile wall in the bathroom and I slammed into the bathtub and lost consciousness. This time I became enraged and empowered; I yelled at him, and I went and told my mom that he had been molesting me. And then we just went on with our day like nothing had happened. We visited Carlsbad Caverns."

They then drove back to Minnesota, and when they arrived her mother immediately called the police and got a restraining order. "I had to do the sexual assault interview, you know, demonstrate on a doll, all of that," Philomena recalled. "It was my first interaction with the criminal legal field." Because she didn't want to testify in court, her stepfather was able to plead to child assault and not a sexual charge. She had "a tremendous amount of guilt about that," which stayed with her for a long time. And she has struggled with PTSD and back pain from the assaults.

After the restraining order, Philomena began to see a psychologist. "I remember our first visits," she said. "I would just go there and go to sleep. I slept a lot in middle school, because I couldn't sleep when my stepfather was there. He would come into my room and I was scared. So, I had hypervigilance suicidality."

Self-harm became "a way of life, beginning around age twelve," she said. "I like to cut, you know. At one point I took a whole bunch of Tylenol and passed out—actually, I never told anybody about that. By sixteen, I was doing a lot of drugs, and I liked to drink vodka, straight, until I couldn't taste it. In order to survive, I had to compartmentalize. So, there were parts of me that had to be completely walled off. And they were very self-destructive parts of myself. And then, they did not always want to be walled off and kept apart. So, they would kind of barge in, and then ruin things in my life. It sounds really weird and crazy, right?"

I assured her it didn't sound weird or crazy at all. It sounded familiar.

"I had parents who were very dysfunctional," she said. "And I had to be an adult, very young. And so I had to become extremely resourceful in getting all of my needs met. And when my mental illness got to a point where I needed to get help, I would query the people around me and find the resources that I needed. I think part of that is a function of having an alcoholic parent, and then part of it is just living in America, right? That's how we have to function as people. We're only able to survive insofar as we can muster up the resources to get to the next level of care, right?"

At the height of Philomena's alcohol and marijuana use, her

mother discovered that she had stolen her grandmother's ceremonial pipe and was using it to get high. Her family was terribly upset, but that did not stop her substance use. Finally, when she was a junior in high school, her mother insisted she go for residential care for alcohol. "My mom was just tired of it," she recalled. "Because she saw me as somebody who had a lot of potential, she got to a point where she was just going to throw me out. So, at seventeen, it was either go to treatment or be homeless." She spent forty-five days in a residential program in Blaine, north of Minneapolis—beginning on April 1, 1995, still her sobriety date (or in twelve-step parlance, her "birthday")—and then three months in a halfway house before returning home for her senior year of high school while attending twelve-step meetings.

She continued with talk therapy but was suspicious of mental health medications, largely because twelve-step meetings at that time actively discouraged any psychiatric meds and medication-assisted substance use disorder treatment as simply substitute addictions.

"My dad needs to be on medication for his bipolar disorder, I know this," she said. "And I really believe in medication. Like, all I want is for the people in my community to have access to Suboxone, and to get on Suboxone, so they can stop dying, right? I'm a huge advocate for medication . . . for *other people.* I just have kind of a mental block when it comes to myself. I've had some success with Buspar [buspirone, a common antianxiety medicine], which I was given in college for anxiety—and again in law school, although I think everybody needs to go on meds in law school—and I liked it. At some point I got a diagnosis of OCD, and I took something for that. But I just feel I have this weird relationship with drugs. It's a little bit of cognitive dissonance that I might have with myself."

She has powerfully mixed feelings about twelve-step meetings, too—even though she recognizes they saved her. "Look, part of me feels traditional AA is a cult at this point," she said. "And, apologies to anyone who's a member of AA, but I feel like it can be very unscientific, and problematic on many levels. But it's also a part of who I am. I went to meetings for about twenty years."

I told her I understood—while I am endlessly grateful to AA and its long, powerful tradition of peer support, there is a reason I found myself gravitating toward twelve-step groups that did not discourage medication use, and also did not require complete secrecy and anonymity. I think part of the challenge for all of us in recovery, and all of us being treated for mental illness, is figuring out how to support (or at least not disparage) all evidence-based approaches, including the ones that didn't work for us, those that *did* work for us but we've moved on from, and those that are currently working for us—all as a way of backing a sort of mental health "pluralism." It's similar, in some ways, to believing in your own religion (or your right to not believe) but supporting the rights of others to believe in their religions.

After graduating from the University of Minnesota with a double major in political science and American Indian Studies, Philomena tried to figure out what to do with her life. She was working at the Birchbark Books store—owned by well-known author Louise Erdrich—and attending meetings, including the Thursday Central Pacific meeting. One night she was sitting at home wondering about her future when she heard a voice say to her, "Talk to a lawyer." She didn't know why.

Not long after, she was at a meeting and got to talking to Mark Gardner, a scrappy, gregarious solo practitioner family lawyer, twenty years her senior, who seemed to know everyone in AA in greater Minneapolis and was a sponsor to many. (Gardner was also quietly part of the mental health world—he was being treated for bipolar disorder and had grown up with a father who was director of research at the famed Menninger Clinic in Kansas, once a mental health mecca.) She told him about what the voice said. And without a moment's hesitation, he said, "Come work for me. I practice family law, and you'll be helping people right away. I've got a roster of women from foreign countries who are getting the shit beat out of them and losing their kids. Addicts trying to get their kids back. I mean, it's human rights law—just very, very applied. We don't write fancy papers. We go to court."

She started working in his office, which already had two other assistants—who, she learned, only got paid if they brought in family law cases that came to fruition and the firm got its fee. The assistants soon quit, and Philomena took over running the office, overseeing cases in Mark's name, and studying for the LSAT. She got into the University of Minnesota Law School in Minneapolis, where she did well, and she clerked for a judge in the Mille Lacs Band Tribal Court as well as for the county public defender's office in Minneapolis.

During her first summer in law school, she found herself in an intense conversation with a friend about her continued guilt over stealing her grandmother's pipe. The friend suggested she make a commitment to amends, including participation in the "Sun Dance," a multiday Plains Indian ritual.

"I had to do some hard stuff to make up for that," she told me. "I made a commitment to amends, including sun dancing on a reservation in South Dakota for several years. It's a really strenuous four-day ceremony in the peak of summer, so it's hours and hours of dancing in the hot sun, really sacrificing your body. Many different religions have things like this, a way of reconnecting the spirit, getting into a flow. But it wasn't physically easy."

PHILOMENA GOT MARRIED and had a daughter during her third year of law school, who her mother helped her raise after she and her husband split. She graduated in 2008, right in the middle of the financial crisis, and got a job as a clerk for a Minnesota state court judge.

After two years there, she was hired for the job she thought would change her life, working for a prestigious Washington nonprofit, the Indian Law Resource Center. One of the first projects she worked on was lobbying the U.S. government to adopt the United Nations Declaration on the Rights of Indigenous Peoples.

One day Mark Gardner got a call from her at his office.

"Guess what I'm doing?" she said. "I'm calling you from the White House. I am here representing *all the Indigenous people on earth!*"

This was her dream job. She was on the front lines of addressing violence against Native women, international climate funds and their impact on Indigenous peoples, and human rights violations against Indian Nations. Unfortunately, the environment was not ideal for her mental health.

"Within a short time, I started having a lot of anxiety," she said. "It was very hard for me to sleep. I was a single parent raising a three-year-old child without any family or anybody around. And it got to me. Not sleeping was really hard. And because I lived near the Capitol, there were always helicopters going around and sirens going off, and the noise just made me overstimulated all the time."

With the increased stress fueling her PTSD and anxiety came a return of her suicidal ideation, made scarier by the fact that she was no longer responsible for only herself but also her child. She was able to hold herself together at work. "I never lost it, anywhere," she said.

"I'm not a public losing-it kind of person. In fact, almost nobody knows about any of this. I have to tell people, and when I do, they don't believe me."

Finally, her supervisor suggested she get help. She was working for Armstrong Wiggins, who had experience with serious trauma himself, having grown up a Miskito Indian leader in Nicaragua, fighting for human rights there and being jailed twice.

"He could tell that something was up," she recalled. "It was probably just my facial expressions and my behavior. I was probably pretty low energy. And it was probably clear that I was going through a depression."

He connected her with a male psychiatrist, who diagnosed her with PTSD and connected her with a female psychotherapist in Georgetown, who she saw for six months and really liked. For the first time in her life, she also actually wanted a psychiatrist to prescribe some medication so she could get more immediate relief. But he was reluctant to do so. At the time, many mental health professionals believed PTSD only responded to talk therapy. (This was 2011, and the field was just starting to accept the use of antidepressants and antipsychotics for PTSD; they are now commonly used.)

"The psychotherapy was amazing," she recalled. "I mean, it was life-changing. But when you just do talk therapy for PTSD, it takes a long goddamn time before you see any results."

When she had first arrived in D.C., Philomena's plan was to work for the Indian Law Resource Center for five years. But, during her second year she started wondering if she needed to live somewhere more conducive to her mental health. The Washington office was a place where Native leaders from all over the country came to plead their local causes. One day, the chairman from the Bad River Band—her family's tribe in Wisconsin—came in to discuss the problem of a proposed open-pit iron mine that was close enough to the headwaters of the Bad River that the reservation's water supply could be endangered. It was a good cause, and a good excuse to leave the pressures of D.C. tribal politics.

She and her daughter moved to northern Wisconsin in the late fall of 2011, and she became a staff attorney for the Bad River Band of the Lake Superior Tribe of Chippewa Indians. The offices were in the tribal town of Odanah, just below the Bad River (and a mile south of where it feeds into Lake Superior), where there were a handful of municipal buildings, a health center, an elderly center, a food distribution center, and, just down the road, the Bad River Lodge and Casino. The reservation itself covers 193 square miles of land along Lake Superior, and it had few full-time inhabitants until the late 1980s, when federal support increased and the Indian Gaming Regulatory Act allowed the casino to be built in the early '90s. Today just over fifteen hundred people live on the reservation itself, but it straddles two counties to the south (including Ashland, where Philomena lives), with a combined population of over 20,000, who can all access everything from harm reduction to walleye fishing (since the reservation has the main walleye hatchery for the area).

Philomena dove headfirst into blocking the mine and succeeded. She then began using her state and federal contacts to work on child welfare matters, tribal self-determination issues, and environmental causes.

After three years as a staff attorney for the tribe, she moved to a different job in the same building, as an attorney and policy analyst for the Great Lakes Indian Fish and Wildlife Commission. There she helped implement the tribe's off-reservation rights to hunt and fish, she got involved in the management of wolves and chronic wasting disease, she worked in food regulation and developed a model food code to help sell treaty-harvested foods, and she also did grant-writing and communications and oversaw the grants when they came in. It was a demanding full-time job, on top of which she also decided to do something to stop the shocking rise in opiate overdoses and deaths.

She and an activist who grew up on the reservation created the Gwayakobimaadiziwin Bad River Needle Exchange, a volunteer harm reduction program for the Bad River Reservation and surrounding communities, and raised the money to run it. "I did the grant management, the reporting, all the financial stuff, and the communications," she explained, "plus a lot of direct service. I would take people to the emergency room if they were afraid to go and spend hours there with them. People would come to my house, where I would pack up the kits for folks who were making saves with naloxone."

She worked another twenty hours or more a week on the needle exchange, on top of her full-time job. Besides the direct work, she was also working to create models that might be employed in other, larger tribal communities around the country that were similarly being devastated by opiate addiction.

"She's somebody who could be a national-level superhero," said her mentor Mark Gardner, "but is focusing on where she's from and where she lives."

The harm reduction work wasn't only for tribal members. "We're also serving four counties on a direct basis, so we work with the white people in our communities," she said. "They're part of our community, too. And nobody's taking care of them. So this is part of our Indigenous diplomacy, right? We're a people that have always taken care of our settler communities. We're all very, very connected."

The work was fulfilling but often overwhelming. She and her

partner decided to have a child of their own, a son born in 2015. And then things began getting tense with her boss.

"Without going into a lot of details, I ended up having to quit my job," she told me. "And I loved that job. And I was *really good at it.*"

In September 2021, she went back to working for the tribe, this time as economic development coordinator, overseeing the construction of a new tribal food production facility, working on tribal food insecurity and chronic disease prevention, and also developing a larger harm reduction and overdose prevention program.

As her son began showing signs of learning differences, and her daughter became a teenager struggling with her own anxiety and depression, Philomena felt her own mental health worsening. She was falling into a deepening depression, having suicidal thoughts.

"I have some weird theories about what happened to me and how I'm supposed to process it," she explained. "And this is actually cultural. As Ojibwe, we believe in multidimensional time, right? And my theory is that sometimes when I'm experiencing this emotional turmoil, the purpose is for me to shoot back in time and help the person that I was back then, struggling, so that I actually make it.

"I feel like when this is happening, the veil between time gets really thin, and I can actually go back and help myself."

I was curious. Was this a fairly new idea, or did she actually perceive anything like that coming from the other side when she was younger?

She started nodding her head even as I was finishing the question.

"I don't know," she said. "Although, I literally don't know how I could have survived otherwise. I didn't have hallucinations, visual or auditory, or anything like that. But, now that you ask, I did have a vision of myself. I had a vision of myself in the future. And I wanted myself to be somebody that I could trust, because . . ."—and she started tearing up—"because I *didn't have that,* you know. I was probably in middle school when I started thinking about this stuff. And it was just a concept, you know? I didn't have an idea of what it would look like or anything like that. But . . . someone who could *love me,* right?"

I asked her if she needed a moment. She nodded, stared straight ahead, then slowly picked up a tube of ChapStick and silently applied it to her lips but didn't wipe her eyes. More than ten seconds passed.

"Are you okay to keep going?" I asked.

"Yeah," she said, definitively.

IN MAY 2022, while Philomena was at the annual walk to recognize missing and murdered Indigenous women, she confided in a friend that she was feeling "suicidal all the time." While the feeling wasn't unfamiliar to her, the sheer volume and intensity of the thoughts seemed different.

"A lot of it, I think, had to do with burnout," she said. "I had been doing too much for many years. And this area I work in, overdose prevention, is really hard. All through the pandemic and then after the pandemic, we kept losing people to overdoses. And so, I was just dealing with a lot. I really needed time to process and create some boundaries that were healthy for me." She was able to raise half a million dollars for the harm reduction program, "so we could finally bring on some paid staff to do the work."

She also began teaching Indian Law part-time at the University of Minnesota Duluth and was named a Bloomberg fellow at the Johns Hopkins School of Public Health, which will allow her to pursue an online Doctor of Public Health degree in addiction and overdose prevention. With this degree and her tribal economic development position, she feels she'll be able to innovate locally and nationally to improve mental health and substance use services on reservations. "I would like to explore something like a WPA project or a CCC project for the opioid epidemic—citizen's health care!" she said. "It will include people who have been successfully treated, who sometimes struggle with employment, and are sometimes in the best position to help."

But she has also worked on taking better care of herself. She went to more sweat lodge ceremonies. She even took up sewing—which was something originally introduced into Native cultures by the "boarding schools that were designed to civilize us," she laughed. "But I like it, and being a good seamstress is now something that's valued in our communities. I find it centering."

She also made a change in her medical care. She had been seeing a male psychiatrist she really didn't like, and who she thought talked down to her. So, in midsummer she switched to being cared for by a female psychiatric nurse practitioner at the reservation health center.

The nurse practitioner suggested she try an antidepressant—a type of medication she had always resisted in the past—because the drug was also used to treat sleep disorders. Philomena had no doubt that her sleeping patterns were a disaster. And I'd guess the nurse practitioner didn't care if Philomena mostly saw the medication as being for sleep, as long as she took it.

"So, actually, right now I'm using a Western medicine. It's a sleep medicine that is *awesome*!"

"What is it?" I asked.

"Okay, wait, let me go get it," she said. "Okay, it's called trazodone (Desyrel). It's old-line and was originally used for depression. But it's great for sleep. I love it. I'm a big fan."

Chapter Two

Henry

Henry Platt's first day of freshman orientation at the University of Pennsylvania didn't go as planned.

It was the last week of August 2017 and everything should have unfolded pretty smoothly for Henry, a baby-faced young man with strawberry blond hair, an infectious smile, and a silky-smooth tenor singing voice he couldn't wait to try out for the campus glee and a cappella groups. While the eighteen-year-old had just moved east for the first time after growing up in Los Angeles, he was already comfortable on Penn's West Philadelphia campus. His parents had met there, and three of his older siblings—he was the youngest of five—had gone there.

After a day of orientation sessions, he went out with a group of people he had just met to his first fraternity party. It was crowded and sweaty, and while he wasn't much into the drinking, what got to him more was the endless posing for cell phone pictures and videos. "No meaningful conversations, no true connection," he remembered, "just a sea of intoxicated young adults conducting their own photo shoots." He joined in, becoming "the artistic director of my own photo shoot, staging the perfect shots that feature all my new best friends, with drinks in hand and uncontainable smiles on our faces." And then came all the vibrating notifications from Instagram, Facebook, and Snapchat, as all the moments they had just lived and captured appeared on their feeds, causing them to temporarily stop living in the moment to see how many "likes" they got.

"It felt good to be a part of the crowd," he recalled. But then, after everyone headed home, he sat down in his dorm room, on the fourth floor of Penn's century-old quad, and started to sob.

"I've always been a very sensitive person," Henry told me, "but usually, if tears were shed they were more positive than negative, or in response to an emotional situation that actually warranted it. But these tears were, like, for no reason. They were just because I was, like, *existing*."

It was the beginning of a year in which he struggled to do everything from getting up in the morning to staying alive. And it just so happened that his struggle took place as Penn, like many universities, was being forced to confront just how outdated and inadequate its campus mental health care was. Henry found this out very quickly. As his crying continued, on and off, for weeks, he called his mother and they decided he should immediately go for an emergency mental health session at Penn's Counseling and Psychological Services—which everyone called CAPS.

But it was a Saturday. And, at that time, CAPS was *closed on the weekends*.

"The weekends were the hardest time for me, the most unstructured time with the most social pressure going on," he recalled. "They were, like, terrifying. So, when I heard they were closed I was completely shocked."

They decided to bypass the student health system, even though his parents were paying for it, and instead found a private doctor immediately who they would pay out of pocket. And they couldn't help but wonder what happened to all the students who couldn't afford that.

This was just the beginning of Henry's care, which ended up intertwined with the litany of larger mental health controversies at Penn, as well as many colleges and universities across the country.

A week after the first day of orientation, a Penn senior took his own life, after a long battle with depression; he was a former president of one of the Jewish fraternities on campus, and since Henry was Jewish, active at synagogue and summer camp, the death particularly resonated. It was the fourteenth reported suicide of a Penn student in the past four years. It wouldn't be the last. And Henry, even while struggling with his own health, would try to find a way to do something about that.

TODAY, HENRY PLATT lives in New York City, where the twenty-four-year-old works by day at Warner Chappell, the publishing arm of Warner Music Group, and by night he performs, solo and in groups. He has a substantial following for his singing on Instagram and TikTok.

But Henry easily flashes back to his fraught freshman year in college and the people who helped him through his mental health crisis. The luckiest thing that happened to him was that a young woman named Hannah Lottenberg—who was also from L.A. and attended the same Jewish summer camp he had, although they hadn't ever been friends before—was also a freshman at Penn. They were thrown into the same freshman seminar. And just a few days into the semester, they found themselves with a group of students, wandering west on Walnut Street toward a party, when Henry pulled Hannah aside and said out loud, for the first time, "I have depression."

"I don't know how he knew that he could trust me, and I don't know how we made such an instant, literally *insane* connection," Hannah told me. "But we will be best friends forever because of that."

Henry was very clear on what his relationship with Hannah meant to him: "I don't know if I would have survived the year if she wasn't there."

I have often heard stories about that "freshman friend," who basically saves the life of a person they just met in a new school. I've also heard too many stories of people who were not lucky enough to make that unique connection in time. So, I was interested to learn more about their courageous friendship—the courage of Henry to trust, the courage of Hannah to take on such mature responsibilities for a new friend at the age of eighteen.

Classes began that year on Monday, August 28. Several days later, Henry tried out for Penn Counterparts, the campus a cappella group, and looked gleeful in the Facebook announcement that he had been one of only three Counterparts "newbies" selected. But it wasn't long before he found himself having a hard time getting up in the morning—and the more unstructured weekends were particularly challenging. He tried to keep his distress and dysfunction a secret from everyone but Hannah, and he got pretty good at pretending everything was okay.

"When I got to college, it was the first time I was existing outside of the context of my family, and sort of starting with a clean slate," he said. "At first, I thought it would be very freeing to have the room to just be who I am. But I think I had no idea who that really was. So, I found the transition very, very difficult."

Part of this was his being more open about "my queerness. I knew from a very young age, but I wasn't open about it at all, even in high school. When I got to college, it was the first time I was trying to be out, and open about my sexuality. I just didn't know how, exactly. And this really was taking a toll on me." It was especially challenging because, to Henry, everyone at Penn looked as if they had it more together than he did. "I felt like I was surrounded by so many people who, well, you know, Penn's a very professional place."

Over the past several years, there had been discussion on many university campuses about the demand to be—or at least appear—completely together, unflappable. At Stanford, this student state of collectedness was referred to as "Duck Syndrome," since a duck appears to effortlessly glide across the surface, while paddling frantically underwater. Unfortunately for the University of Pennsylvania, their version of the phenomenon got a catchier nickname, "Penn Face," which received national attention after being covered prominently in *The New York Times*—and then tied in the press to the school's suicide statistics.

All of this pressure on students was exacerbated by the internet: "Social media adds a whole new element of difficulty when you're in a new social environment," Henry said. "It all piled up." He found himself checking his Instagram at least once an hour, "just to see what I had missed and to check in on my 'likes.' I searched for external validation, believing that if my photo were to hit a certain threshold of likes or comments, it would mean that I had worth. Looking back, it seems hilarious that I would think it to be so important. I envy my parents who grew up without social media. They didn't have to worry about what everyone else was doing at all times. They could focus on their own experiences, be present in their conversations, establish stronger connections, and, most importantly, speak openly."

Singing remained Henry's favorite release, but he had one unique thing to deal with on that front. He wasn't always sure if people were being nice to him because they liked him and his singing or if they were impressed that his older brother was Ben Platt—who was currently on Broadway and had just won a Tony for his lead role in *Dear Evan Hansen,* a musical that explored teen suicide, depression, and social anxiety.

Henry grew up in Los Angeles in the public eye. His father, Marc, is a major stage and movie producer (*Wicked, Legally Blonde*) and his mother, Julie, after a successful career in banking, became a major Jewish philanthropist and a longtime member of Penn's board of trustees. (Henry's parents were college classmates of my co-author, which is how I met him.)

I told Henry I knew something about this myself, growing up the youngest child in a high-profile family, especially following my older brother, Teddy, who was famous from the time he was twelve, when his battle with bone cancer, which caused him to lose his lower right leg, was international news. A lot of younger siblings have birth-order issues; it's not unusual. But I completely understood that when Henry was struggling with depression, being Ben Platt's kid brother didn't always help.

"There was a part of me, when I was very unmotivated, just feeling like I didn't know why I was getting out of bed every day, and then I see my brother who was, like, being so successful," he recalled. "And I was kind of resentful of that, in a way. I talked to my therapist about it and, it's very interesting, I think in therapy, through my tools, I have learned to really just be proud and embrace all of who he is and what he's done. But I think when I was feeling so down on myself, I skewed all of his successes in a negative light."

HENRY'S MENTAL HEALTH got worse over that first semester. This was true even after his psychiatrist started him on the antidepressant sertraline (Zoloft) and continued to meet with him for talk therapy once or twice a week. Henry missed classes; he had to force himself to eat and lost weight. His roommate, Adam, was helpful, but eventually Hannah decided to change dorms to a new room on Henry's floor, just to keep an eye on him. She got to know Henry's parents and siblings, who would reach out to her when they couldn't get him to respond to phone calls, emails, or texts, which was often. He would do the same thing to her, to the point where she had to threaten to call 911 if he didn't respond.

In late October, to cheer Henry up, Hannah and another friend, Joelle, made a half-hour video, shot all over campus, which began by asking a variety of people what made a good friend ("gives really good hugs") and concluded that all these attributes were true of Henry Platt. This was followed by in-depth testimonials, meant for Henry to watch when he was feeling depressed and unloved, about all the ways he was, in fact, loved—and also how many other people were struggling, too. When they shared the video with Henry's mom—who had, so many times, resisted the temptation to just jump on a plane from Los Angeles to be with him—she was overwhelmed.

"A Mom hopes and dreams for their child to be seen and to be loved—especially when this Mom sends her baby across the country," she wrote after watching it. "I could never have dreamed how challenging these past eight weeks would be for my son, but there is no question that he is blessed and he is cared for and he is loved—what a gift to Henry, to me, to his Dad, and to his whole family. This film is the most moving reflection of friendship I have ever seen and I am eternally grateful."

Besides all the other pressures of college and life, exacerbated by social media, Henry realized that another thing impacting his depression was much more elemental: light. Growing up in California, he had never been in the East when, suddenly, the days got darker much earlier because of the end of daylight saving time. The weekend the clocks were changed was Penn Homecoming, and his sister came to town to check up on him. He had lunch with her, but then went back to his room and refused to attend the football game with his friends or meet up with them afterward.

"I urged him to come," Hannah recalled. "All of our friends were going, and he just said to me, 'I can't handle it.'"

Soon after, Penn Counterparts had its first performance of the year. It was a big enough deal that his parents and his brother Jonah (also an actor and singer) came in to see the show. Henry got to do his first college solo, performing the song "Attention" by Charlie Puth and singing backup on several others. But, as Hannah remembered, "he looked down and depressed. I remember at one point his mom looked over at me and said, 'Henry does not look like himself.'"

And when his friends wanted him to go to the afterparty, he had already left and run back to his dorm room. Hannah called him, "and all he said was, 'I'm just feeling too down, I can't do it. I can't celebrate.' Depression just infiltrates so many parts of your life."

THE SPECTER OF suicide was painfully present at Penn that fall and winter. While CAPS finally did add some weekend hours on Saturdays, there was a general complaint that it still took a long time to get an actual mental health appointment. The administration was being criticized for not making enough improvements in care and for not notifying students and faculty quickly enough when there was a tragedy.

And there were more tragedies. A thirty-year-old veterinary student died, then a thirty-one-year-old law student died, with neither cause of death fully explained. Then the recently appointed chairman of the dental school's department of periodontics took his own life, at the age of fifty. And more people nationally were learning about the university's mental health challenges from a recent *New York Times* bestselling book about the death by suicide, two years earlier, of an outstanding female track star at Penn. It wasn't necessarily that the school had a bigger suicide problem than any other big university, but that's how it was perceived in the media and on campus. Many felt Penn wasn't doing enough to change that perception. It was a uniquely difficult time to be a Penn freshman with major depression.

"I definitely had some suicidal ideation," Henry recalled, "and I was open about it, expressed it to my parents. It never was like, 'Okay, this is my plan, this is how I'm going to carry it out.' I think I was just so overwhelmed with the depths of my sadness, that it sort of felt like the only way to channel it was to say, 'I might as well just kill myself,' or 'I don't want to be here anymore.'

"It was a lot of mind games with myself, to get myself in situations where I could sort of be rescued as a way of proving that, like, I actually did have worth, or did actually mean something to people. If I thought about wanting to die, it would be a lot about wishing I could understand how people would react in the aftermath. I would envision a lot how people would react to the news, if they found out that I was dead, as a way of, like, validating my current existence. And I think a lot of those thought processes were very sick."

ON ONE PARTICULARLY bad night, Henry recalled, "my psychiatrist had called my friend, Hannah—who I had known for only, like, two months. And she was told, 'You have to stay with him all night tonight. Otherwise, I need to admit him to the hospital because I'm worried that he'll hurt himself.'"

Hannah, who was deeply involved in the Penn dance community, remembered getting this call at a rehearsal. She quickly picked up her stuff and went to Henry's room, where they slept together in his bed, staying up nostalgically watching YouTube compilations of Vines (extremely short videos, kind of a precursor to TikTok, for which the app had recently closed down).

"We made it through the night," she recalled, "and I think it's funny because I look back on that and I wonder, like, how did I not freak out? How did I not question, like, what I was doing, and just do it? I didn't think twice about telling the psychiatrist that I was okay with that. I didn't know how. I was so confident, freshman year, that I could take it on." (She did know one reason for her unusual confidence: she had survived Hodgkin's lymphoma in tenth grade.)

I asked Hannah if they told her it was a "suicide watch."

"The terminology was more just 'making sure he was safe,'" she recalled. "I think if I had heard 'suicide watch,' a very scary term, I'm not sure what I would have thought. But I will say that by this time, part of the trust Henry and I had built was that we promised each other, and he promised me, that if he was ever having 'scary thoughts'—that's what we called them, 'scary thoughts'—he would have to tell me."

They even developed their own shorthand language to verify Henry was telling the truth about the severity of his symptoms. "It's actually funny," Hannah told me. "We invented a term to make sure he didn't lie. In his family they use the phrase 'word of honor, WOH.' So, we created one of our own. It was called, and I know it's kind of dumb, HHSSS, which stands for 'Hen-Han Super-Secret Swear.' So, I'd ask if he was having scary thoughts, and he'd say 'no,' and I'd be, like, 'HHSSS.' And he would say, 'Okay, fine, I am.' You don't lie on HHSSS. It would be the *biggest* violation of our friendship."

Whenever he could, Henry let Hannah know how much she was appreciated. "This weekend was one of the lowest points of my life," he told her in an email, "and for some reason you decided to take it upon yourself and help me. Nothing else was helping, talking to anybody else in the world seemed like such an effort, but when I saw you and hugged you and talked to you, it felt like a burden had been lifted off my shoulders . . . You are the world's most beautiful person. Your soul is one of true goodness and you have the ability to impact and better the lives of every single person you encounter . . . Although I can't be the friend you truly deserve right now, I hope you know just how much I love you and how utterly grateful and thankful I feel to have your friendship and support."

JUST BEFORE THANKSGIVING break, Henry's brother Ben was making his final performance on Broadway in *Dear Evan Hansen*.

"For his last show, there was a party afterward, and so my whole family had flown out," Henry recalled. "But my parents wouldn't let me go to the actual show. So I had to just meet up with them later, because they were, like, 'It's too intense for you to see right now.' I had seen it before, but I kind of agreed with them. It was too intense for me right then."

Henry somehow was able to finish up his classes, and when he got back to Los Angeles for break, he spent much of his time in his room. When he joined the family for meals, he seldom even spoke.

The struggle with depression continued when Henry returned to campus. He continued seeing his psychiatrist for talk therapy and medication, and they tried several different medications to see if they would help: the anti-anxiety medicine clonazepam (Klonopin), which made him feel even more reclusive and disconnected. He tried the antipsychotic aripiprazole (Abilify), which caused weight gain, so he was weaned off that.

He had already lived through enough cycles of his depression and anxiety that he developed different coping strategies for different severities of symptoms. He figured out when he could handle things with his local psychiatrist and Hannah, when he needed to call his parents, and even which of his parents to call.

"If I wasn't in a hysterical situation, but I just couldn't get out of bed, I'd talk to my mom," he explained. "She's more of an emotional person, she can understand and talk me through it. But when I was at a ten, and just sobbing or having a big anxiety moment, I knew if I called my mom, it might make things worse. I would be able to feel her worry and her concern through the phone, and we would just fuel each other rather than calming me down. So, for big, explosive moments, my dad would usually be the first phone call, because he could help get me down from the ledge of a ten, and get me down to a five and help me work through it."

While there were still too many days during his second semester when he had trouble getting out of bed, he was able to keep up in his classes, and he became more active in Penn Counterparts, even accompanying the group on its annual spring break performing trip, this year to Dublin.

As so much of his life was revolving around his mental health, he found himself reading more and more about the complaints of students regarding the ease and availability of care, and the pressures students in treatment felt to take medical leaves, from which it could be difficult to return. (As was true at other universities, some felt Penn too strongly encouraged medical leaves for fear of additional suicides on its watch.) There had been a lot of talk from the administration about new wellness initiatives but not much in the way of change.

Just after spring break, Henry and Hannah both received emails from Penn president Amy Gutmann, inviting them, and a small group of other students, to an "informal lunch and conversation" at the president's house. The lunch took place on a Friday in early April, and the student guests represented many corners of Penn life. The two of them were there representing the performing arts, the singing and dancing communities. At one point during the meal, the president announced that she wanted to go around the room and have each student talk a little bit about their experience on campus and where they would like to see Penn improve. Football players wanted more athletic equipment; student government representatives wanted more of a say in policy.

When she got to Henry, instead of talking about the needs of a cappella singers, he immediately launched into a critique of the way mental health care was being handled by the university.

"I remember I sort of went on this long tangent about my experience. I literally laid it all on the table," he told me. "I really talked about how I was frustrated with the lack of access and was feeling that I was not supported throughout my freshman year by the institution. I was lucky enough to have friends and resources outside of the Penn sphere that were able to get me through it. I talked about the wellness efforts, which, while there were some on campus, they were not well-coordinated and not publicized enough."

"I do remember how brave it was," Hannah said. "I also remember being a little bit taken aback: like, how did he have the guts to say that? Then, everyone was kind of looking at each other. Because, mental health is one of those things that everybody experiences but nobody talks about. And you just have to have somebody in the room to *say it.*"

"I wasn't trying to be confrontational," Henry said. "I wasn't, like, being angry. But I was just really speaking from the heart and being truthful. And I think it really sparked something in her because not long after, the provost of our school was asking me to meet him. And I went into his office and he said, 'We are going to create a new position at Penn called the Chief Wellness Officer, who would be a medical professional in charge of overseeing and coordinating all wellness efforts across students and faculty, making sure there is alignment with student health services and the physical health side of things. And we want you to be on a search committee.'"

While Henry's impassioned speech had made an impact, his cause was assisted four days later when Penn was hit with a high-profile lawsuit by the parents of a junior in the Wharton School of Business who had taken her own life two years earlier. According to the suit (which Penn later settled), she had told multiple caregivers in Student Health and CAPS that she was contemplating suicide, but her family believed not enough action was taken to make sure she was safe.

Two weeks after the suit was filed, Penn's president sent an email to all students and faculty announcing the creation of the new "Chief Wellness Officer," and the reorganization of health services so that Student Health, the counseling service CAPS, and the Office of Alcohol and Other Drug Program Initiatives would be coordinated by the new office of Student Wellness Services.

Over that summer, Henry was on the panel that interviewed candidates remotely. He was home in Los Angeles, working as an intern for Universal Music Group. He also started working with a licensed clinical social worker in Los Angeles. She took over his talk therapy, while the psychiatrist in Philadelphia continued to write his prescriptions. This is a fairly common arrangement; some patients get talk therapy and medication from a psychiatrist—who is trained in both—but most do not, often for financial reasons. Psychologists and clinical social workers, who are generally less expensive than MDs, can't write prescriptions, and they specialize in talk therapy. Ultimately, regardless of training, the challenge is to find a care provider with whom you develop a therapeutic relationship, and whose approach appeals to you. Henry's new therapist specialized in cognitive behavioral therapy, or CBT, the most popular form of talk therapy in the world, which focuses less on replaying the past than identifying "automatic negative thoughts" that hamper the present, as well as strategies to keep them from overwhelming or holding you back. (Henry didn't realize until I told him that CBT was first developed at Penn in the 1960s and 1970s, not far from his freshman dorm, by my late friend Dr. Aaron "Tim" Beck.)

Hoping the worst was behind him, Henry put on his brave Penn Face and signed up for more classes than necessary, to test himself. This just caused more pressure. Luckily, because Penn had appointed that new wellness officer who Henry had helped choose—Benoit Dube, a psychiatrist already teaching in the med school—students were being encouraged to share their mental health challenges if they needed to miss a class, get an extension on an assignment, or even drop a course.

Henry found himself using that option the morning of the midterm in his History of the Middle East class. At 9:51 A.M., just before the exam, he emailed his academic adviser.

"As you may know I am currently enrolled in 5 classes, one of which is History of the Middle East. I really believed that I could handle the load of five classes, but as the midterm for this class approached, I became incredibly overwhelmed. Unfortunately, I have been struggling with my mental health, and today, just before the midterm I reached my breaking point." He asked if she could help him withdraw from the class, which he successfully did (but it still showed up on his transcript).

Henry's mental health continued to slowly improve, and he learned better coping skills for when he had breakthrough depression symptoms. The summer after his sophomore year he worked as an intern at NBCUniversal TV Music Services. And then in the fall of 2019, Henry's junior year, he returned to campus where the Penn Wellness program was taking a dramatic step forward. They had recently hired a new high-profile director for CAPS, the student counseling service: Dr. Gregory Eells, a psychologist who had run the same department at Cornell for over a decade. Eells was starting his first full semester at Penn and was to be the face of its deepening commitment to improving student mental health and preventing suicide. Henry was looking forward to working with Eells.

Henry had also, as part of his involvement with the Student Wellness Advisory Group, developed a session on "Penn Face" that was added to the Penn Arts freshman orientation, with the kinds of discussions and materials he wished someone had given him as a freshman.

Then, on a Monday morning, just twelve days after the beginning of classes, a stunning report reached the campus. Dr. Gregory Eells, the new head of CAPS, had taken his own life.

"I remember hearing the news," Henry said, "and, I mean, how could there be any more red flags as to the state of wellness, in general and at Penn, if the leader of its counseling services was struggling so much. It was really surreal."

That fall, Henry got into his first relationship since coming out. He and Hannah worked on making their friendship a little more balanced and less about emergency caregiving: Hannah had been diagnosed with bipolar disorder at the end of freshman year and needed help herself.

Henry also decided to write about his depression—and his anger at the impact of social media—for a new website his cousin had started, called The Conversationalist. He described his "baby step" in the "marathonic journey of mental wellness" and also made a pitch to ban all "likes" on Instagram. The piece ended:

> Someone once told me, "If you aren't yourself, you are robbing the world of something it desperately needs."
>
> So it is time, my friends.
> Start the conversations.
> Check in with yourself.
> Check in with those around you.
> Open up.
> Be authentic.
> Express.
> Challenge.
> Question.
> Cry.
> Laugh.
> Feel.
> That's how we run the marathon of life.

The piece went viral, especially after his rabbi in L.A. posted it on his very active social media accounts. It was soon reprinted in the *Jewish Journal* of Los Angeles.

Henry was feeling better, and even when he wasn't, he was coping more successfully. He was excited to be voted music director of Penn

Counterparts and was put in charge of organizing the a cappella group's spring performance trip, for which they were constantly rehearsing. He was also voted chair of the A Cappella Council, which oversaw Penn's fifteen different specialized a cappella groups. (Hannah was voted chair of the Dance Arts Council.)

They were going to go to London—all the performances were arranged; Henry had been involved with booking all the flights and the hotels. And then COVID hit. And for the first time since he arrived at Penn, Henry was actually feeling sad for a "good reason," a completely external reason. The Penn campus was shut down, the Penn Counterparts trip was canceled, and Henry moved back home.

"So, now at least I'm justified for feeling that there's no reason to get out of bed," he laughed. "But it was really hard. I had all the usual triggers, like not having a structure, plus the feeling of being robbed of a college experience that I really needed and wanted."

One of the only highlights of the spring was that Henry and his two brothers were invited to perform for *Graduate Together: America Honors the High School Class of 2020,* the virtual commencement celebration that LeBron James and others created for all the seniors who were being deprived of ceremonies: it aired live on ABC, CBS, NBC, FOX, and all major social media platforms. Ben, Jonah, and Henry had been singing together since they were all young—there are YouTube videos of them going back to when Ben was first breaking through and Henry was fourteen, and they had just done a recorded performance for Israeli Independence Day of "Ahavat Olam" that was going viral. But this was the first time they had performed together on a global stage. Among the other performers were Pharrell Williams, Bad Bunny, Dave Matthews, and the Jonas Brothers, actors Kevin Hart, Julianne Moore, and Olivia Wilde; even Barack Obama. The Brothers Platt, as they called themselves, did a tasty mash-up medley, with Henry soloing first, then Ben and then Jonah, ending with them all crooning the chorus from a Green Day hit, "Good Riddance (Time of Your Life)." The show was viewed live by nearly 15 million households.

And then Henry went back to COVID life. He did a summer internship remotely from his bedroom. And then, even though it was unclear whether Penn would have in-person classes for the fall of 2020, he and Hannah decided to take a road trip from L.A. back to Philly for their senior year. When they arrived and moved back into an off-campus apartment, Penn announced it would be virtual for another semester—so they stayed and took their classes on Zoom in the apartment. (He also appeared that fall on an episode of the short-lived Netflix reality sing-off show *Sing On* but did not win.)

In December he was home, and his synagogue, Sinai Temple, decided to devote its annual Hanukkah celebration to mental health, in collaboration with the local chapter of the National Alliance on Mental Illness (NAMI). Among the talks by clergy members and musical performances during the hourlong virtual event were actress and congregant Mayim Bialik talking about mental health advocacy and miracles, and then Henry talking candidly about his own mental health. Standing in his parents' bedroom speaking into a video camera, he told parts of his own story and used the themes of the holiday to explore how people can get through the darkness and to the light. Then he performed the song "Beautiful City" from *Godspell.*

When school began in January 2021, with classes still online, the COVID vaccine was finally starting to be administered and there was suddenly, actually, a chance that Henry would get one more normal semester at college—and maybe even an in-person last Counterparts performance. The group was allowed to rehearse in person, but only outside, in a secluded Penn parking lot, still masked. Ultimately the group did not get to perform live. Henry had to do his last solo of college, to an arrangement he did of "Somewhere over the Rainbow," virtually.

But he also realized, as his senior year was ending, that he had made real progress in treating his depression.

I asked him how he thought COVID had ultimately impacted his own mental health and that of his generation of college students.

"It was very challenging," he told me. "But in a weird way, I think there was something . . . and, look, I don't want to, like, try and glorify the COVID experience, because it was pretty terrible. But if there was one good thing about it, it was that a lot of people's struggles were exposed, or they had to sort of come to the surface. There was a union, everyone was experiencing the struggle very *clearly*. So there was a certain feeling of 'Okay, we can have more open conversations with people about how much the world sucks right now.'"

So much has been said about a dramatic increase in mental health problems during COVID. But Henry was suggesting something different: maybe the experience just made people more open because they were more pissed off about the baseline amount of mental illness we just ignore, or underplay, or deny.

"I think it's probably a combination of the two things, for sure," Henry said. "I think on the one hand, maybe for some people COVID was the straw that broke the camel's back, just like going to college was for me, the thing that made me admit I'm actually struggling and I can't pretend anymore. But I also think that when just about everyone is experiencing anxiety—it's, like, the cultural Zeitgeist—then people react to the common experience. And it makes them just open up about it more."

After graduation in 2021, Henry and Hannah took a trip to Spain, and then ended up as roommates in an apartment in New York, where Henry also started dating "my now boyfriend." They both settled into life in the entry-level job world: Hannah at a strategic media-buying and planning firm, Henry in the music industry, while also trying to make it as a singer and contributing to mental health advocacy.

Henry worked first for Broadway producer Vivek Tiwary, known for *Jagged Little Pill* and *American Idiot,* and then he moved to music publishing giant Warner Chappell, where he worked to get the company's songs used in films, television, theater, and other nontraditional platforms, and also to develop brand partnerships that helped songs and songwriters find new audiences.

At the same time, he was learning more about the business of singing and the journey of trying to make your love your vocation—just as his older brothers had. He began performing regularly, solo and in groups, at the Manhattan cabaret 54 Below. And the social media "likes" that so plagued him as a depressed college freshman became something he had a new appreciation for as his "side passion" for singing gained momentum on TikTok, Instagram, and YouTube.

In a unique mash-up of social media ingenuity and subtle mental health advocacy, Henry is best known on social media for a bunch of very short videos that are now collected under the hashtag "Bored Riffing." For those who knew about his depression, they were particularly intriguing. The first ones showed a snippet of some incredible riff by a singer, and then Henry copying it—but, while lying in bed, draped over a couch, lying on the floor, or some other hiding-at-home position from which beautiful singing seemed as if it might be challenging. As the short videos progressed, he would sometimes appear sideways on a pillow in a complete funk or waking up from a sound sleep and just riffing. Some of these "Bored Riffing" videos have over three million views.

Henry's health has been relatively stable since he moved to New York, but he has recently decided to make a few changes. While he still takes Zoloft for depression, as well as a blood pressure medication, his physician recently added a prescription for the antianxiety agent lorazepam (Ativan). He had taken the medication before but never had an Ativan prescription for more than a small number of pills during a very specific challenging time, which he could take when he felt his anxiety triggering. Ever since experiencing a bad bout of COVID in 2022, he feels that he overreacts to symptoms of illness.

"My physical health anxiety has gotten really bad," he explained. "If I feel like I'm getting sick, it's too easy to convince myself it's something far worse than it is." It has happened often enough that he and his physician agreed he should have Ativan with him and not have to wait for a new, small prescription. "I carry some in my backpack now," he said. "The knowledge that it's there gives me a little comfort. And when I need it, I take it."

He also decided to look into changing therapists for the first time since the summer after his freshman year in college. He wondered if he "needed a fresh set of eyes in my life." Many times, when people decide they have outgrown their therapists, they just stop getting talk therapy—which can be okay for some people and disastrous for others. While some people stop because of finances, others stop because they simply don't know how to find another caregiver and can't conceive of starting a new relationship of such medical intimacy.

But Henry knew he wanted to try a new therapist, perhaps someone more local with more experience with LGBTQ+ patients. He did some online research and found someone. They worked together for a few months, but ultimately he decided to return to his original therapist—but with the fresh perspective of a twenty-four-year-old working in New York.

Besides work and therapy, Henry has been performing and also trying to write more of his own songs. He has started one that explores his mental health journey.

"It's sort of about that element of self-sabotage and how it relates to depression," he explained. "Even though we rationally know what's best for us, it's so easy to get into a spiral of self-sabotage. While very specific to my depressed experience, I think it's very common. In small ways and big ways, I think everyone has a sort of inner saboteur."

What do you call it?

"Right now, it's called 'My Sabotage,'" he said, "but it's still coming together."

Chapter Three

Gabrielle

Gabrielle Anwar has played a lot of roles in her long and intense public life. She began as "that girl" in a Paul McCartney video and a BBC series in 1986 at the age of fifteen, when she was still at London's Italia Conti Academy of Theatre Arts; she appeared on British TV shows, made a Hollywood splash on horseback starring in the 1991 Disney drama *Wild Hearts Can't Be Broken,* but then got more attention for her smaller, stunning role the next year as Al Pacino's tango partner in Oscar-winning *Scent of a Woman.* She went on to make many movies and TV films, had a starring role in *The Tudors,* and then spent seven years as the star of the USA Network spy drama series, *Burn Notice,* set in Miami where she now lives.

But her most important role is one she has never really talked about before: "Bipolar Mom" is how she described herself to me.

"Actually, Bipolar Mom who was good enough at acting that nobody knew I was a bipolar mom." Except her three kids, especially her firstborn, Willow, who she was pregnant with at the 1993 Academy Awards, had when she was twenty-three, and grew up through her mother's stormy moods and addictions.

In fact, Gabrielle herself didn't truly understand she was bipolar and what that meant for nearly two decades, until she fell in love in her early forties with Miami hospitality entrepreneur and financial investor Shareef Malnik. He was introduced to her symptoms on a date in Martha's Vineyard, when he suggested maybe she shouldn't have another drink—and she punched him in the face.

While he realized then and there she needed help—which she denied as she had to others before him—he also began wrestling with whether a person in love can demand that another get help. He told her he didn't think they could get married until she got proper medical care. But he wasn't sure he would hold her to that.

"What I finally realized," he told me, "was that I loved a woman saddled with this debilitating mental illness, and I loved her more than I loved my own personal comfort, and that my commitment was to her, no matter what."

So, after years of all kinds of personal journeying—through Veuve Cliquot and stimulants, through eating and sexual disorders, through misdiagnoses by Hollywood doctors who prescribed her stimulants (which she happily took because they made her *more* manic), and through every kind of alternative therapy, cleanse, fast, and meditation—Gabrielle Anwar finally agreed to try the one thing she had spent her entire adult life avoiding at all costs. She committed herself to more traditional evidence-based psychiatric medication to stabilize her volatile moods, combined with aggressive personal, couples, and family talk therapy.

For the past ten years, her life has been considerably different. Better. Calmer. Safer.

Gabrielle Anwar was born in England in 1970, the second child of an industry couple: her mother is British film and TV actress

Shirley Hills, and her father is Indian-born film editor and producer Tariq Anwar (whose father was an Indian Muslim film performer and whose mother came from a Jewish family in Austria). She grew up in a tiny village on the River Thames, about twenty miles outside of London. Her mom retired from acting after having Gabrielle (in part, she told me, because of postpartum depression), and her father worked several jobs at the BBC to support the family (he would later become an Oscar-nominated film editor, for his work on *American Beauty* and *The King's Speech,* among others).

Her mental wellness journey began fairly early. Starting at the age of four, Gabrielle recalled being sexually touched by a man next door, who she later came to understand was on the autism spectrum. Her parents realized this was going on because she would pull up her dress in public and do other things suggesting premature sexualization, but they declined to pursue charges. Gabrielle said she remembered the man as "an avid whistler, so my body would turn inside out when I heard whistling."

She first got her period at age eleven and started having mood instability, although, she joked, "it may have just been the rage of realizing you're going to have your period." This is when she started lashing out—literally, she sometimes hit her mom.

"I would just rage at my mother," she said. "And my mother would rage back. We just went for each other's throats. We matched each other's vehemency." She was taken to a psychologist to discuss her periodic rage. "He had me do a bunch of exercises," she recalled, "and he did age-appropriate psychological testing. He didn't seem to think there was anything wrong other than preteen angst." There was no additional treatment, and it wasn't until she was thirteen that it was clear there was a diagnosable problem.

There was a boy in the school she had a crush on, and she found out that another girl had been with him—supposedly in sexual ways Gabrielle wasn't "in any way ready for." She became so jealous and upset that she went into a girls' bathroom and started writing in black Magic Marker that the girl was "a slut" on every possible surface: "any piece of wall, on the toilet paper, in the toilet bowl, on the doors. I wrote it psychotically about two thousand times." She recalled being taken to the headmistress's office, where she had her period, and was "bleeding all over my school uniform . . . they wouldn't let me go to the lady's loo." When they finally let her go, she was a mess.

"The next day," she said, "if I had any blood left in my body, I would have slit my wrists rather than go back to school." Of course, on the way to school, she ran into the girl whose name she had written all over the bathroom, who was not only angry but much bigger than she was. She punched Gabrielle in the face, breaking her nose and knocking her to the ground, and like a scene from some bad teen movie, other students gathered around, chanting her attacker's name and goading her on. After being taken to the emergency room, Gabrielle went immediately home. And she barely left the house again for the next year. She developed agoraphobia, and her face was also disfigured—and couldn't be repaired surgically until the swelling went down. So her mother, who had recently gone back to college to get a teaching degree, decided to homeschool her.

To get her through that difficult year at home, Gabrielle's mother switched from normal school lessons to teaching her Shakespeare, singing, ballet, and even tap dancing. After recovering from facial surgery, she auditioned for the school her mom had attended, Italia Conti Academy of Theatre Arts—the British prep school of stars, where many of the students had been stage-mothered since birth. To her surprise, she got in.

Students at the school were often hired to play young people in

British TV productions and onstage. So, she started getting experience.

She also started getting more manic. She was cutting herself, drinking too much, and generally starving herself so she could remain skinny. While she was developing as an actress, her best acting job was pretending, while working, that she was otherwise okay.

"I had stored in me so much trauma that the director would say 'Action!' and out would come the trauma," she recalled. "Away from work, I would get triggered by jealousy or some teenage romantic faux pas and I would go ballistic, and I would have what you would now describe as a psychotic break—regularly. Screaming rage, exhaustive ranting until I would literally collapse in a heap in the corner of a room, shaking and then just catatonic."

When she was eighteen, she overdosed on her mother's muscle relaxants and was found by her brother, passed out in the kitchen. She was taken to the hospital, released, and soon back to work.

During this time, she met and fell for an American actor ten years her senior, Craig Sheffer, who she first encountered in the cafeteria at Pinewood Studios in England, where he was making a movie and she was working on a children's TV series set at a school newspaper called *Press Gang.* They began "an extremely passionate and tumultuous relationship" that unfolded, on and off as well as long-distance when they were working, over the next few years, fueled by a lot of dramas, disorders, and mutual triggering.

The stories of what was happening behind the scenes make the seamless performances in the movies they were both churning out during that time even more surprising.

During one of the couple's frequent breakups, Anwar was living in the Venice Beach apartment of her high school friend Emily Lloyd, while Lloyd was in Montana playing Sheffer's girlfriend in *A River*

Runs Through It. Ironically, while that film centered on the drinking and gambling addiction of the brother played by Brad Pitt—which led to that character's murder—Lloyd would later recount in her own memoir that she had, by then, been diagnosed with a form of schizophrenia, a psychotic illness (which is different from a mood disorder like depression or bipolar, because a main symptom is disordered thinking, not feeling). She had her psychiatrist on call on the *River* set with director Robert Redford's blessing.

After Emily returned from making the film, she and Gabrielle rented a house in Laurel Canyon. "It was oddly enlightening living with Emily," Gabrielle recalled, "because I was in trouble, but compared to where she was, I was the sensible roommate." With all the parties at the house and their work schedules, the place was a disaster. "I was fastidious with OCD," she recalled. "Emily's OCD, unfortunately, did not include housekeeping. Once, Steven Spielberg telephoned for her. I answered the phone but immediately dropped it, as hundreds of ants came spewing from the sticky receiver."

It was Sheffer who insisted she go for her first-ever inpatient care at Sierra Tucson. At one point he proposed to her, and then rescinded the proposal until she went and got help—which triggered her to cheat on him and make things worse.

Gabrielle's six weeks at Sierra Tucson were eye-opening. She did several different kinds of therapies to explore the roots of her addictive behaviors. She had signed up for the eating disorder program because it was the only one with an opening when she was available to go. But she learned a lot about her use of alcohol and her violent lashing out. And she got a chance to focus on hypersexuality in the Sex and Love Addicts Anonymous meetings, where she wasn't the only well-known actor.

I told Gabrielle I thought sex addiction might be the most

underappreciated aspect of mental health and addiction. I honestly think this is the biggest taboo in mental health these days—the last thing people will admit to but, with internet porn, the one that's probably most pervasive. It's a huge issue, among a lot of people in recovery from drugs and alcohol.

"You're absolutely right," she said. "Until then I just hadn't been paying attention to it as an addiction. In my relationship with Craig there were long periods when I didn't do anything sexually that was detrimental. But then when he un-proposed, I said, 'Fuck you. You don't want to marry me, after all!' So, I went viral. I went *sexually* viral."

ONE THING SHE tried to address at Sierra Tucson was her long history of self-harm. She had done a good bit of cutting on her wrists and arms. "I just wear a lot of bracelets," she said, "because I have a lot of scars." But there was one thing she had never admitted to anyone.

Before she told me, she paused for a second. "Okay, I'm going to say something that's very delicate."

I reminded her that she had already shared a lot that was delicate.

"Well, I'm very embarrassed by this."

I told her I understood and was honored that she was willing to be this open.

"Okay . . . so I had to have a physical examination when I was there, and I was really glad that the one place they wouldn't look was where I did the most destruction."

But then she got caught. "I had a lot of blood under my fingernails," she recalled, "and one of the therapists was astute enough to say, 'What's that about?' And I cursed myself, but I just said, 'I've been scratching myself.'"

The therapist looked puzzled. "Well, we don't see any signs of it on your physical exam."

And Gabrielle said, "Well that's because I scratch my anus. So you wouldn't have seen it."

Gabrielle has always been grateful that the therapist didn't overreact. "She was very good. Her poker face was fabulous. So, I didn't feel as dirty . . . well, I did feel dirty, I felt terribly dirty. But at least she didn't make me feel worse. They changed my medication and made me cut my fingernails down so I couldn't cause any more trauma to the area."

SHE LEARNED A LOT during her inpatient stay. But she also gained five pounds, which her doctor probably loved but she couldn't stand. As soon as she got out, she was starving herself again. And then, she took a job filming an Italian TV series in Rome, for which her voice was going to be dubbed in Italian.

"It was a disastrous production, and during it I discovered cocaine," she recalled. "I was going a little cuckoo. I was twenty then. In the morning I was playing a thirteen-year-old character who was getting raped. And in the evening, by the time we were done shooting for the day, I was the thirty-year-old version of that character who'd had five children and wanted to become a nun. The content was so ludicrous." And triggering. Before leaving the United States, she had been dating a musician, and one day she saw in the tabloids that he was "cheating on me with Madonna." She said she went out with a bartender from the place the cast frequented; she did too much cocaine with him, and the bartender raped her.

Three weeks later, she realized she was pregnant, for the first time ever. She immediately decided to quit the production—without telling anyone—get on a plane back to London, and have an abortion

"I was pregnant and high as a kite," she recalled, "but I got home." An old boyfriend took her to get the abortion. The production company sued her, and she believes this is the first time her agent and her attorney saw any big red flags about her health and welfare. "There were some rumblings on my team, and I was thinking 'Oh, I better get my shit together.'" But she didn't. She was, however, able to keep this quiet, even after returning to Hollywood. One night, when she was in a very dark place, she cut her wrist with a Swiss Army knife. She recalled a friend from London who was with her, Kelly Marcel (then a rising actress and later a well-known film writer), called 911. After being stitched up, Gabrielle checked herself into a hospital psychiatric ward for treatment but checked herself out the next day.

I asked her if she ever got flagged by the companies insuring the productions she was in, and if she had taken steps to keep her treatment secret—like not letting her medical insurance pay (when it would). She said she didn't recall any problems like that.

She played many roles during this time, including the scenes of her dancing with Al Pacino in the Pierre Hotel ballroom in *Scent of a Woman*.

What finally ended this spiral of illness was that she got pregnant again—she had sex once with a would-be film producer and realized she was pregnant on her twenty-third birthday, in February 1993. She kept it quiet while in Austria filming a Disney remake of *The Three Musketeers*. But during the Oscar ceremony that spring—when *Scent of a Woman* had five Academy Award nominations, and Pacino won for Best Actor, which otherwise would have propelled her career to a whole new level—she confided in director Martin Brest that she was pregnant. "I remember his face falling," she recalled. "Another one bites the dust."

But she couldn't have been happier. Even though he wasn't the father, and they technically had broken up, Craig wanted to help her raise the baby.

And, as is true for many women with psychiatric and neurological conditions, pregnancy made her feel much better, healthier. With the pregnancy came a wash of hormones that, however temporarily, seemed to alleviate her cycling mania and depression and her desire for self-medication. It made her even more interested in naturopathic health care—meditation, yoga, cleanses.

"I had never been so happy, never felt so stable," she recalled. "I loved my body, understood my body for the first time. And I felt connected to other people."

She went into labor during the November 1993 premiere of *The Three Musketeers,* feeling her first contractions as she "waddled" down the red carpet. She remembers Willow's birth as "my rebirth. I always say that my baby gave birth to me." Afterward, she experienced none of the postpartum depression her mother had with her. She felt amazing, and breastfeeding allowed her to maintain that healthy feeling for the better part of a year.

"I stopped nursing only because Willow was done," she recalled. "I would have continued because I felt so great. I would have continued nursing her until today," she said with a laugh, "and she's almost thirty."

Within days of the end of lactation, "I felt this dark, dark, dark shroud take over me and I fell. I just fell into the abyss. At one point I was holding Willow and I took a kitchen knife out of the holder and I said to Craig, 'I can't, I can't . . . I *just can't* do this.' And he was like, 'Well, who are you going to kill? Me, Willow, or yourself?' And

I was so confused by the question that he called the hospital, and I checked myself in and said I would do whatever I needed to do to never let Willow see me holding a knife again."

She was in the hospital for several days. A doctor diagnosed her with bipolar disorder and put her on the initial medication usually used for that illness—the mood stabilizer lithium (Eskalith), as well as the stimulant dextroamphetamine/amphetamine (Adderall), which can help with the sedation that lithium often causes, especially as patients are adjusting doses. He also connected her with a psychotherapist.

Unfortunately, as soon as her lithium dose stabilized, Gabrielle decided she didn't like the sedation it caused. She only wanted to take the stimulant. So, for years, she filled her prescriptions for both medications—but she only *took* the Adderall. Instead of stabilizing her mood, she was deliberately elevating it.

Today, presumably, both a physician and a patient would be more careful about this—especially with the lithium, since it works in a narrower therapeutic range than most medicines and is one of the few common treatments for which blood levels are supposed to be checked at least a few times a year. Gabrielle may have gotten away with this for so long because she was a celebrity and traveling so much for work. But there have always been people who are prescribed psychiatric medication—especially by primary care physicians—for whom refills are a little more automatic than they should be. Things have changed somewhat in the past few years as the opiate crisis reminded doctors and patients how casually medicines are sometimes prescribed. But it remains a little too easy to hide from a busy physician.

Craig stayed in Gabrielle and Willow's lives but they never married. "We were very sexy," she said, "but, my God, we couldn't do the laundry!" She and Willow lived in a small house in Topanga Canyon. The one connection she maintained to mental health care was a psychotherapist with whom she formed a solid relationship. She would take little Willow to the sessions with her. And while the sessions and the relationship were helpful, she now regrets some of the things her young daughter went through because of her illness.

"I think most of the effects that I had on Willow in her early childhood came from me being this speeding mother," she said. "I still had that aggression, I still had that rage, but I would utilize it in life. I would drive too fast. And Willow would say, 'Mommy slow down.' Or, you know, I would go through a red light and Willow would say, 'Mommy you went through a red light.' And I'd be like, 'Ehhhh. No, I didn't, Mommy didn't do that!'"

Her hypersexuality was "off the charts. Here I am with a toddler, and I was just sleeping with *everybody*."

There were times when she felt "indestructible . . . I could learn my script, the dialogue in my script in a day for a whole episode. There was nothing I couldn't do." But she found herself turning down the more ambitious work.

"My film career had come to a crashing halt," she said. "I turned down some epic roles during the first few years after Willow's birth, *Legends of the Fall, Little Women, Shakespeare in Love* . . . I chose smaller roles in smaller films that would better serve a schedule with a baby. I was not confident enough to bite off more than I could chew, and raising Willow was all-consuming. I wasn't on the cover of *Vanity Fair* clasping my swollen belly and breasts; therefore I was cast out into the no-man's-land of tarnished ingenues who refused to play the fame game. My agent had predicted this, which is why he tried to talk me into terminating my pregnancy [with Willow]. So, I fired him."

Over the next few years, Gabrielle married actor John Verea, and they had two children, a son, Hugo, and a daughter, Paisley. She went through the same cycles of relative stability during pregnancy and breastfeeding, and then falling off a mental health cliff again afterward. "I was still really cycling, really fluctuating," she recalled, "raging at my husband, trying to conceal it from the children, making it up in other ways to the children by being supermom and super happy and just super. I must have been scary. I had that sort of expression painted on my face whenever I was with my children because I didn't want them to know what was really going on."

She was determined to be a better mom and explored a number of approaches. Most intriguing was the work of Hungarian pediatrician Emmi Pikler, who developed ideas on infant freedom of movement and interaction while studying life in orphanages after World War II. Piklerian parenting involves an attempt to give children as much freedom as possible without putting them in danger, so they can learn problem-solving skills. Gabrielle became a "Piklerite mom."

After divorcing Verea, she raised her three children by herself, but with assistance from Craig Sheffer—who Willow considered her father, and the other two considered their godfather—especially when she was traveling for work. It wasn't always easy.

"I realize Willow and Craig have their own prognosis of my bipolar influence on Willow, and I probably wouldn't disagree," she told me. "Craig and I were very angry with each other, each blaming the other for the degeneration of our love. We both made the intractable mistake of showing this pain to Willow. I haven't vomited my acrimony all over Willow. But it was my responsibility to vaccinate her against all contamination, and in an attempt at natural medicine, I have failed."

As the kids got older, she started working more, playing a regular character on *The Tudors,* and then taking a full-time television job as the female lead in the USA Network spy series *Burn Notice,* for which she moved to Miami, where it was set.

For the first several years of the show, she was still taking prescription stimulants and remaining slightly buzzed all the time. "I was really trying to find my footing as the character, and I was on my best behavior," she said, "but I was still ordering copious amounts of champagne and putting it on USA's bill."

SHE MET HER future husband, Shareef Malnik, at a dinner under the stars at an organic farm in Homestead, south of the city. Shareef's family is prominent in Miami, best known for their landmark restaurant, The Forge. Shareef had been in the hospitality business most of his life, until moving into financial investing; he has been most visibly active philanthropically in Make-a-Wish Southern Florida, where he is chairman emeritus but still chairs the capital campaign and the annual fundraising ball. He had been married several times and was known as an extreme sports aficionado and something of a thrill-seeker. He was fifty-one when they met; she was thirty-nine.

"I was really quite naïve with regard to having any true understanding about mental illness, until I met Gabrielle," Shareef told me. "I recognized the fact that I would meet people throughout my life that I felt could possibly be mentally ill, but I didn't know anything about it. I didn't know how to interact with it."

They dated for several months before he realized he would need to learn. They went away to Martha's Vineyard, and one night were out to dinner with friends they were staying with, remaining in the bar afterward on their own. "We were doing some tequila shots," he recalled. "And I said something to her, like, 'I don't think you should have any more tequila shots, you know?' And she said, 'What about you?' I told her I was fine—I'm twice her size—but I was just afraid that she was getting really wasted, you know.

"So, she hauled off and punched me in the face. And I was in total shock. Being somewhat inebriated myself, I tried to make a joke: 'Well, you hit me on my right side. Why don't you just go ahead and hit me on the other side.' So, she hauled off and punched me again!"

They went back to their guest room in the friends' house, "and she's screaming at me at the top of her lungs. And I'm like, 'Oh my God, I don't even know how to respond.' I just thought, 'Wow, this is just not typical behavior from someone I've been getting along with so well,'" he said. "Finally, she goes to sleep. We woke up the next day, she was fine. But she wasn't apologetic at all. She just said, 'Don't ever tell me that.' And I wrote it off to having a bad reaction from alcohol."

But as the days and weeks went by, he got the impression that this woman he was falling in love with had "been on her best behavior up to that point, but that night may have cracked the door open for her to be more outrageous and aggressive in her communications and behavior toward me," he explained. There were episodes not fueled by any alcohol, and she was talking about this voice in her head, which she explained "is not really a voice, but it's this dark thing. And it's real. And it's telling me bad things. You know, and it's telling me how bad you are."

He wondered then—and still wonders today—if she has control over what she does. "She says she doesn't, because of her bipolar disorder. And I feel that she does have control over what she does, but she chooses to behave certain ways with certain people. For example, she's not going to haul off and punch her daughter in the face. She doesn't agree with me about this, we talk about it often, but I believe you're not going after everybody in that restaurant, you're gonna go after the person who is *not going to leave you.* It's a weird paradox, I feel secure with you so I can go after you, I can show you the worst side of who I am, like my darkest, darkest moments."

He finally told her that if she didn't get help, it could be a deal-breaker for their relationship. He researched specialists and it turned out one of the best-known psychiatrists in the country was there at the University of Miami.

IN THE SMALL WORLD of mental health advocacy, I've known her doctor, Charles Nemeroff, for years. And "Charlie," as he is known—he's now chair of psychiatry at the University of Texas (UT) in Austin—got permission from Gabrielle and Shareef to speak with me.

"Gaby came to me depressed, morbidly depressed," Charlie recalled, "and the question was, What was the diagnosis? It took some time in getting a history and realizing that she was clearly bipolar. And she was *not happy* with the diagnosis [which she had heard before]. She was also extremely anti-medication. This is part of the Hollywood set, the notion that, you know, natural medicine is good, medications are bad."

They had a "friendly disagreement" about how she should be treated. "Sometimes people have to get worse before they're willing to accept treatment," he recalled. "And we went through a lot of ups and downs, literally, until she was willing to accept lithium as an important medication. And then we switched her to a combination of medications that have led her to be pretty stable."

But he wanted to make it clear that it wasn't the medicine alone that helped. People too often underestimate the importance of a therapeutic relationship—not only to create a consistent, dependable place to share challenges and concerns but as a key to staying on medication. I told him that was a lesson I had learned many times myself.

"I believe this about all my patients, but particularly for Gabrielle. The cornerstone of helping her get better was the relationship we had together," he said. "I did my best to respect her boundaries and allow her to trust me, which is a big issue for her with men. And she wasn't getting any special treatment because of who she was. Her billings all went through regular commercial medical insurance."

I was surprised to learn she used traditional health insurance to pay for her treatment. I've known public people who seek out psychiatrists and psychotherapists who don't take insurance, to keep their care more hidden from potential employers. Insurance still carries a high deductible for therapy (so each session can cost over $100 out of pocket). But Nemeroff and I are in agreement that a big "problem in American society" is the large number of mental health providers who don't take commercial insurance and "insist on cash only." I do understand this is partly because private and public insurance reimbursements are too low, but the result is that almost half of the world of talk therapy is largely unmonitored and understudied.

BOTH GABRIELLE AND SHAREEF wanted to better understand why she suffers the way she does. "Well, she had a lot of early trauma," Charlie explained, and "the data would suggest that if you're genetically vulnerable to a major psychiatric disorder, and you're exposed to early life maltreatment, you're more likely to develop a major psychiatric disorder, and the course of the disorder is going to be more pernicious. In bipolar disorder, the episodes of depression and mania are going to have an earlier age of onset, and they're going to last longer. You're also more likely to develop comorbid [simultaneously occurring] disorders, like PTSD, ADHD, and anxiety disorders. And you're more likely to have suicidal thoughts and to attempt suicide. And then on top of that, you're less likely to respond to evidence-based treatments. And you're less likely to accept them. It just makes everything worse."

While he questioned Gabrielle's previous treatment, she, clearly, hadn't always followed previous doctors' orders. It's important to understand all the reasons previous treatment may not have worked. For patients and their current treatment professionals, it's sometimes a little too easy to dismiss everyone and everything that came before. So-called gold-standard treatments—individual medications and "cocktails"—do change with advancing research. And with many psychiatric disorders, and especially bipolar disorder, up to half of those diagnosed stop taking their medications and reject their diagnoses. It often takes far too long, with risky medical trial and error, before they can accept and embrace the diagnosis—and the process of staying current on treatments.

"One of Gabrielle's greatest concerns—and this is a theme for people with bipolar disorder—is that she did not want her artistic creativity to be curtailed. We had endless conversations about that," Nemeroff said.

Most of her issues were ones that almost everybody who gets diagnosed with bipolar disorder has—and thinks are unique to them (which is, in fact, part of the illness). But some also did have to do with being an actress. "Gabrielle suffered from what many women in Hollywood suffer from—you get to a certain age and you get discarded," he said. "I know of one incident in which she was offered a part if she'd sleep with the producer, and she refused and didn't get the part."

When Gabrielle started treatment with Nemeroff, and she and Shareef did counseling with him together, they weren't yet married. It took a while before the sessions left Shareef with optimism.

"She would turn on me in the therapy session," Shareef recalled. "Suddenly, it's all about me, everything that's wrong with me. Right? She completely manipulated the whole concept of getting better. And I am just getting annihilated. And it's embarrassing. So now I feel like I'm defending myself. And all I'm trying to do is help her."

He wanted to marry her, but he also wondered if they should wait until her symptoms were under better control. "My plan was to marry her, and quite frankly, things were not resolved when I asked her to marry me," he said. "But I wasn't going to abandon her when she needed me. And this was going to take a really big transformation for me as a human being because, honestly, I don't think I ever understood that high level of commitment. And maybe that's why she's in my life, for me to rise above my own self-indulgence and selfishness."

I told Shareef I was really moved by what he was saying. The fear of being rejected, I said, is so primordial when you have one of these illnesses. One of the biggest issues for people like me is this: Can we talk about our illnesses and still be loved? The fact that you're able to love someone in spite of their illness—to not see them *as* their illness—is a beautiful thing. I know it doesn't always work out that way for people. It's so hard to know: Am I safe with the people around me? How did you talk to Gabrielle about that?

"Well, I shared it with her, a lot, that I'm not going to abandon her," he said. "But at the same time, Charlie said something in one of our sessions that I thought was really powerful. He said, 'Mental illness is not an excuse for bad behavior.' So don't take advantage of me. I'm holding you to a high standard of behavior in spite of your mental illness. You don't have carte blanche to abuse me because you know I'm not going to leave you. So we're going to have to put on our big boy and big girl pants here, and have a lot of integrity with each other in order to make this work."

He also got involved with her medication—and the way couples deal with each other's medications could fill an entire marital medical manual. Asking a spouse or partner if they took their meds can be interpreted, at any given time, as a helpful reminder, an unwanted intrusion, even a judgmental criticism. If a significant other understands the illness and how symptoms can slowly kindle, they might recognize or be concerned about changes before the person with the illness. But noting that isn't always welcome (especially in bipolar disorder, since the first symptoms are often low-level or *hypo*mania, which feels good).

"Gabrielle hated it so much when I suggested she might be 'cycling,' which is a perfectly accurate word for this, that she finally asked me to stop using the word," he joked. "She did have a code word, however, for when she recognized she was struggling and wanted me to be super-understanding to avert a total meltdown. She called that darkness 'The Joker.'"

He is doing his best to understand the love/hate relationship people have with any medication for a chronic illness, but especially mental health meds. "It has taken her a long time to even accept the idea that she will most likely be medicated for the rest of her life," he explained. "It's not worth *not* being medicated. Every time people start feeling better, they want to get off their meds because they feel good enough. It's a crazy paradox. Once you get off your meds, of course, you need to get back on the meds again. And, so she's finally at the point where, while she can be a little unpredictable sometimes, she realizes that this is her life and she's appreciative of medication that works."

Still, he said, you never know how a random conversation with someone who doesn't know any better can challenge the delicate med balance. "One time we had these people over to the house," Shareef explained. "We were on the board of this think tank, and I notice Gabrielle is having this intense discussion with one of the board members. I asked what was going on, and she said, 'Oh, he told me some of my weight gain is because of my medication.'

"Everybody thinks they know enough. And, of course, she's still looking for that silver bullet that makes it so she doesn't have to take the meds. I just thought, 'That is so irresponsible. Does he know what you do when you're off your meds?' No, of course not. And does he have to live with it?"

GABRIELLE SAID IT took about two years of work in psychotherapy and adjustment of meds before she really felt stable. "It changed my life," she said, "and it changed my husband's life because we wouldn't have had a life together for sure without it. And, it changed my children's lives. My youngest children don't really remember me being psychotic, but Willow does. And I think to this day, Willow doesn't want to truly embrace my stability, for fear that it isn't as stable as she might believe. Because she was so traumatized in her childhood by me, by my bipolar disorder, I think she still struggles to embrace the stable mother that I've become." (I did reach out to Willow to request an interview for the book, but she declined.)

Gabrielle's treatment was interrupted by going off her meds so she and Shareef could try to add to their family through IVF. She had three children, two still living with them, and he had a grown son, and a grandson, but they hoped for a child of their own.

"In the midst of the IVF, I was in a horrendous downward cycle," she recalled. "Once the children were in bed, I called Shareef at his restaurant and told him he better come home immediately or else. When he arrived, I was on the floor of our bedroom, in a puddle of tears, shaking uncontrollably. When he tried to comfort me, I refused to let him touch me and raged at him with vicious accusations and vulgarity, trying to punch, slap, scratch, bite my husband. I had these manic episodes often, for many years, but this time, Shareef telephoned the fertility doctor in Los Angeles. She suggested he administer a quarter of the teeny estrogen pill I had in my regimen of hormonal drugs for the cycle. Within fifteen minutes, I was completely normal. A little puffy, and red, and terribly sore, but utterly relaxed, calm, and embarrassed. I couldn't undo the damage I had caused, or unsay the hateful words I had screamed, but I was no longer in pain.

"We did not get pregnant. And I think Shareef was thoroughly relieved. And we carried on, I, in a state of remorse and shame, and Shareef in a state of apprehension. I would have, like a lot of women struggling with infertility, done anything to fulfill this destiny. But the darkness of bipolar disorder destroyed my competency. I frightened my quiescent baby daddy, and I frightened myself. Back on my meds, I can be a stable, balanced mom to the children I am already blessed with."

She's still a very active seeker. She directed and starred in a provocative and funny film, *Sexology,* in which she and friend Catherine Oxenberg traveled the globe in search of sex experts to help them have better orgasms.

And one of the last times I spoke to her, she explained that she and her oldest daughter, Willow, were doing a new treatment together to try to break down some family tensions: what she called a "plant-based medicine adventure" overseen by a couple of psychologists "who look like Joseph and Mary." It began with a twenty-four-hour "guided infusion" with the psychedelic mescaline to "open things up."

Personal and "guided" use of substances with psychedelic properties—some plant-based, others synthetic, and even some FDA-approved medications—has been done in Western medicine since the 1960s. But they have become more popular and more commercial in the past few years, with very little regulation. Even the prescription medicines, such as ketamine (a dissociative anesthetic used mostly in pediatric and veterinary care and a common party drug), are often being used in "off-label" infusions, and the uninsured sessions are paid for out-of-pocket. This is sometimes done in conjunction with more traditional mental health treatment—especially for patients with treatment-resistant PTSD and depression—other times as a temporary substitute, occasionally as a wished-for "cure." Some hope "microdosing" of psychedelics could augment or replace traditional psychiatric meds.

Gabrielle was clearly just trying this on the side. She hadn't even told her psychiatrist before doing it. "Charlie doesn't know about it," she said with a grin.

I found this sort of funny, because I knew from talking to Charlie Nemeroff that he had started a small center at UT to study psychedelic use for PTSD, depression, and anxiety, but only under the supervision of a medical team. He had introduced us to another patient who he had helped try ketamine, unsuccessfully, for her lifelong depression. But he did see promise in "this whole emerging area about the use of psychedelics. Of course, the data is still pretty meager. And we're trying to put some scientific rigor to it. But we have seen some life-changing experiences."

Gabrielle and her daughter did a series of sessions with mescaline, followed by regular family therapy sessions without mescaline, all on Zoom. They seemed useful if not life-altering.

But, whatever her journeys, she takes her daily medications—currently the mood-stabilizing antipsychotic lurasidone (Latuda) as well as venlafaxine (Effexor), which is used to treat depression, as well as anxiety and panic disorders—and she does so religiously.

"I will never stop taking this medicine," she said. "It has saved my life. If I stop, I am my own burden, and I know the consequences in my life."

Chapter Four

—

Miss Tonie

When Tonie Dreher counsels recently arrested New Yorkers who hope to be diverted to supportive psychiatric care instead of jail at Rikers Island, or people just out of prison with mental health and addiction problems, she lets them know she understands what they are going through all too well.

"They say, 'Oh, Miss Tonie,' and I say, 'Okay, I'm telling you, Miss Tonie has been some places, and Miss Tonie has seen some things,'" she said, with a knowing grin.

Tonie, a self-described "big person" in her early fifties with a big personality and a sly sense of humor, also lets them know how much has changed since she went into recovery from crack cocaine addiction in her early forties in New York City—after more than twenty years of active using and selling, dozens of arrests, and painfully losing children to social services.

"Things are not like they used to be," she told me. "People really play with your life now. They are purposely, intentionally putting in fentanyl. So, you have to be careful."

She also sees the racial realities of addiction changing. "This epidemic is not just striking down Black people anymore. I counsel a lot of white people. And I see, this thing is striking *everyone.* It's not a colored thing. It's not an economic thing. It's not discriminating. People stay stuck on 'white people get better health care than Black people.' That might be true, but little white children have died in the streets from fentanyl just like little Black children. And we have to stop putting this thing in a color scheme, because it doesn't have a color choice."

The biggest problem she sees, and she does everything she can to remedy by sharing her hard-lived experience with her counseling patients, is something she now knows isn't new or surprising at all—which is why she is frustrated by how few people understand and just how long it took her to understand.

"I wish that people, especially Black people, knew that mental health is a serious issue," she said. "What I learned is that substance abuse was a small part of my problem. The biggest problem for me, the biggest challenge for me, has been mental health. And I didn't even know that I *had* a mental health problem."

Tonie had been given some mental health drugs in prison—fairly arbitrarily, and mostly just to help her sleep. It wasn't until a near-death experience sent her to a year in a New York sober living facility that she started understanding her drug addiction was being driven by intense psychiatric symptoms: paranoia, mania, psychosis, and abuse flashbacks.

And it was only because she was lucky enough that when she applied for public assistance so she could stop selling crack—and selling herself—the therapist who was supposed to see her for ten minutes for an intake interview took a unique interest in her case. She not only built a long therapeutic relationship with him through talk therapy—still going on after more than a decade—but he helped her get and stay on the proper medication and get peer support to stay sober. She has been diagnosed with schizophrenia, paranoid type, manic depression, and PTSD.

Tonie now earns a living as a counselor for dozens of New Yorkers, and occasionally gives talks about her own experiences to mental health professionals in training, who don't know nearly enough about the challenges of what is called "carceral" care—the treatment needed, but not often enough received, before, during, and after incarceration. She has become friends with one of the nation's experts and innovators in such care, Dr. Elizabeth Ford at Columbia, the former chief of psychiatry at Rikers Island (who introduced Tonie to me). But she has never shared her full story before. And it's a tale still unfolding.

Part of her journey now is reconnecting with all of her children, some of whom were raised by relatives (and always thought she was their aunt) and some of whom went into foster care or adoption. She isn't exactly sure how many there are. One of her children set up a private Facebook group so the others can connect and communicate.

"I've run into so many *me's*," she said, "who have lived the exact same story as mine, people who don't know mental health is something you can talk about and not be ashamed of. For most of my life, I knew nothing about mental health."

TONIE DREHER WAS BORN in 1968 and raised in rural Lexington, South Carolina, living with her mother and younger brothers in a small house across the street from their family home where her grandmother and other relatives lived. The adult members of the family worked on a nearby vegetable farm. When she was young, her stepfather would often lock her mother, her younger brother, and Tonie in a closet while he was at work—with just some food and a porcelain potty—because he was so paranoid about being cheated on. He would also periodically disappear, which she later was told was because he suffered from mental illness and was being hospitalized. As soon as Tonie was old enough, she was enlisted to help take care of her younger brothers—there were eventually six of them.

She recalled being physically abused as a child, often hit or beaten. She also recalled being molested by an older man in the neighborhood at an early age, and she later came to associate these events with times when the family didn't have enough money to pay bills; she recalled the man sending her home afterward with money. She said her mother, who is still alive but from whom she is estranged, has denied this ever happened.

"She's my mom," Tonie said with a shrug. "I let her live in whatever world she wants to live in."

What everyone agreed upon, however, was the event that forever changed Tonie's life. When she was eleven, she was watching her younger brothers when she had one of them cross the street, while she watched him, so he could borrow a hot hair-straightening comb. Her cousin, who had the device, was then supposed to walk the boy back across the street. While washing a sink full of dishes, Tonie heard "a loud commotion in front of our house." Her brother had tried to cross the street by himself and was hit by a car and killed. Her mother blamed her—she blamed herself—"and so that was yet another burden I carried." Unfortunately, this led to more physical abuse.

"Some days when I shower, I still see the scars that were small when I was small and are big now that I'm an adult," she said, "and I'll have an emotional meltdown. I remember all of that."

Not long after her brother's death, she made a suicide attempt. "I took an overdose of pills. And I woke up and I was angry at God because I said I couldn't even *kill myself* right," she said. From then on, "pills were always my source of attempts. And I would always wake up, you know."

Tonie was only able to remain in school through tenth grade, because after that she was taking care of her five remaining brothers. She also got pregnant, by her first boyfriend, at the age of sixteen. She had a daughter and went on to have two other children with him while still a teenager. (Tonie was raised a Jehovah's Witness: she was taught that birth control was okay, but not premarital sex or abortion.)

It did not occur to her until much later in her life that her hypersexuality could be a psychiatric symptom, or that sexual release was one of the few dependable ways to slow down her racing thoughts and her visual and auditory hallucinations.

Her mother then decided she wanted to start her life over and moved to New York City, leaving Tonie's brothers temporarily in her care. In the meantime, Tonie's first boyfriend, who was older, said he thought she needed the opportunity to be a young person again and agreed to raise two of their kids so she could start over herself; her cousin took the third child. She soon was pregnant again, had a daughter with another man, and then got involved with another man who was in the military. She moved with him to Texas with her fourth child, and her brothers moved to New York with their mom.

Then, in her early twenties, Tonie moved to New York too, staying with her mother and brothers in a five-bedroom apartment in the Bronx. She got a job at Wendy's and also worked as a clubhouse security guard at Yankee Stadium, often in the dugout, which she loved.

It was at this time when she began to realize "that there was something not right with my mind." She would "suffer with bouts of depression, but I'm very good at masking, so that's what would always happen. I suffered in silence, because I could put on a face, and no one ever knew what was wrong. But my insides were crushed. I didn't know anything about mental health in those days. No one talked about it."

She then met a woman on the first floor of her mother's building, whose apartment "was known as a crack house, and that's where I had my first experience getting high. And I liked the feeling, I *liked* the feeling, because I didn't have to think about anything. I didn't have to deal with anything or anybody."

At the time, she was also in an abusive relationship, and she had had another baby. "One day I woke up. My boyfriend and I had been arguing," she said. "He attacked me, kicked me in my head with Timberland boots, accused me of cheating . . . I probably was cheating. And after that I just walked away from everything, including my children. My journey to addiction went from there. I became the neighborhood drug dealer, because selling crack was easier than selling my body. And that was my life."

Her mother threw her out, so she lived where she could. She was arrested frequently—over thirty times—for possession, for selling a controlled substance, for drug paraphernalia. She learned about the concept of ATI—"alternatives to incarceration," which were starting to be made available for people whose maximum sentence if convicted would only be a week or two (but who could end up waiting in jail for trial much longer than that). But she recalled ATI rarely being offered to her. And sometimes she thought thirty days in Rikers—where someone else was responsible for feeding her and putting a roof over her head—sounded like "a good break from the streets."

Sometimes at Rikers she would request to stay in the mental health unit. "I didn't think I had mental illness," she explained, "but

I just listened to the other inmates who said if I went there, I could sleep the whole time, and I needed my rest." They gave her meds to help her sleep. (She recalled getting quetiapine—Seroquel—which is a pretty strong antipsychotic to be used primarily to help someone sleep who does not have a psychotic illness diagnosis.) They did tell her she seemed depressed, but she didn't really know what that meant.

"I didn't understand what mental health even was," she said. "People always talked to us about not using, about addiction."

This cycle continued for nearly a decade. Then, in her early thirties, she was arrested and after spending pretrial time at Rikers, accepted a plea agreement for a sentence of two to four years. She was sent to the Albion Correctional Facility, a medium security prison for women west of Rochester near the Canadian border. There she didn't try to stay in the mental health clinic, preferring to live in the general population. But she did get medication, "because it's so readily available in the prisons. All you have to do is go say you're suffering with something. They don't test or diagnose you. I didn't know what my symptoms looked like. I didn't pay attention to the idea I could have a *condition*. The meds made me feel good, helped me sleep. I was high; it was another way of being high."

As she has more recently learned about how jails and prisons can be places where people sometimes get proper mental health care for the first time in their lives, she is angry about what she saw being offered. "There is no therapy in prison for anyone," she said. "Black people, white people, brown people, yellow people, doesn't matter what color you are. No therapy. You see a shrink for maybe five minutes, seven at the most. Then time is up, they call in the next person. It's a medication pipeline. You get diagnosed, but maybe that diagnosis is incorrect. And then they don't tell you that the diagnosis follows you *forever*. And the medications you take stay on your medical records. It's a business: the mental health/incarceration pipeline."

But there were some positive aspects of her first long prison sentence. "Nobody wants to be locked up, told what to do, when you can eat, how long you can shower, when to go to bed," she said. "But I wasn't on the streets. I knew I was gonna sleep at night. I had a boyfriend when I was at prison, so he made sure I was taken care of.

"But I think the most important thing was that I had some peace of mind there. For the first time in a long time, maybe ever, I had an experience of *clarity*, and structure." She also converted from Christianity and became a Muslim in prison, which added to her understanding of her need for structure. Yet she had no doubt what would happen when she got out. "I went there," she said, "to do my time and go the hell home so I could smoke crack."

She was at Albion for four years. Once she got out in 2004, she immediately moved to Harlem and began using and selling crack again. It took another five years before anything changed. She recalled living on benefits from the Temporary Assistance for Needy Families program (TANF, formerly known as "welfare") and the Supplemental Nutrition Assistance Program (SNAP, formerly known as "food stamps"). "Every other week," she said, "a payment for $60.58 would hit the system at midnight and I could take it out of a cash machine, and that was 'get high' money. I never used it for food, never went to buy any female products, just used it to get high." She didn't have a residence; she slept on couches at places where she got high, or places that were abandoned. She tried shelters but they were "definitely not for me." And unless it was too cold, she sometimes slept outside at St. Nicholas Park in Harlem, on a particular green bench at 128th Street and St. Nicholas Terrace.

"I would never lay down," she explained. "It wasn't safe. I would only sleep there sitting up. I was actually in the neighborhood recently and saw my bench. I just had to smile and shake my head, thinking how far I've come from there. But I was on the streets a long time, you know. I see people every day who are homeless. You don't know why they're homeless, why they are out there. You don't know why I was on the park bench. You just would have looked at me and said I was a drug addict. I think that in order for any healing to begin in this country, people have to know the people on these park benches are people."

DURING THIS TIME, she also had several more children; she is not sure how many.

"I was using to live and living to use," she said, "and in between, the children kept coming. I did have times where I had to sleep around in order to be high, with no protection going on or anything." Several of these children were born testing positive for cocaine, so she was encouraged to sign them over to the foster care system. She felt she had no choice at the time.

Just a few weeks after giving birth to a daughter in 2007, she agreed to have her first major inpatient substance use treatment, at the nonprofit Daytop Village Recovery Center in upstate Rhinebeck, New York. She was there for three months but soon after started using again.

Then in March 2009, as she was about to turn forty-one, she had an aha moment.

"Every time that I went to this one old man's house to use," she explained, "he would . . . well, it's called 'blowing your high.' He would always blow my high. He would always make it seem like someone was hiding in one of the rooms, to blow my high.

"I was extremely paranoid in my last days of using and I took a hit of crack there one day. And in my mind, what I saw as a vivid vision was a man walking from around the corner of his kitchen and shooting me. I saw the fire coming from the gun. I saw me dying. I could hear myself screaming. I could hear the old man telling me to shut up, that I had brought it on myself," she recalled. "Everything was so vivid. And I knew in that moment: that's not how I wanted to die. I didn't want anyone going to tell my mom that they found her only daughter dead in a crack house.

"The very next morning, March 17, 2009, early before the building opened, I was standing outside the intake on Third Avenue for Phoenix House in Harlem to go into treatment."

She lived at the Phoenix House on Vernon Avenue in Long Island City for the next year. She only slipped once while living there. She went out on a day pass and went to Harlem hoping to see several of her children who were living with her mother and siblings. Instead, she ended up using. And after hours of getting high, she left the crack house at midnight and went directly to the hospital—what was then called St. Luke's Hospital on 114th Street—and demanded to be committed to the psychiatric ward "because I had to be out of my mind to get six months clean under my belt and then go back to the neighborhood and throw everything away. And I didn't know why. And the doctor came to my room and said, 'We're gonna send you back to your program. This is not a psychotic meltdown. You're just high.'"

So, she was allowed to return to Phoenix House and finish the last six months of her program.

After she got out of Phoenix House, she decided that the only way she could afford to live if she didn't want to go back to selling drugs was to apply for SSI—the Supplemental Security Income for people who are poor or disabled. To qualify, she was told she needed to see a therapist.

"Oh shit, what do I need a therapist for?" she recalled thinking. She was given an appointment at the SSI office on Varick Street in SoHo and was assigned an intake counselor, a psychologist named Paul.

He turned out to be "the beginning of the rest of my life." He has been her therapist ever since, "the longest relationship I've ever been in." Even though he has changed jobs several times, he maintains his therapeutic relationship with her.

At first, she had her doubts. "I mean, here's this white man sitting in front of me, and I'm saying, 'What are you going to be able to tell me about myself? I'm just here to get my social security benefits.' When he started getting close to my surface, close to my truth about my life, I would go out and use, and not show up for appointments. I guess I was running from myself."

I told her I loved that phrase, "close to my surface."

Paul talked to her initially about "not being present" but soon realized that her distraction was far deeper than that—Tonie had been experiencing paranoid delusions for years. She heard voices, she sometimes saw things that were not there.

"They wanted to try to get me on the right medication," she explained, "because they believed I had schizophrenia, as well as suffering from PTSD and depression." At the same time, the therapist had to convince Tonie that she was, in fact, worth treating, worth helping to get better.

"I saw myself as worthless," she said. "That's what I was told my whole life. And when you get this your whole life, you believe it, right? I don't think that I took myself seriously from the time I was a teenager. Who was gonna want a worthless nobody? Who was gonna want to have someone as a girlfriend who wasn't a virgin, who had been molested? Who was gonna want somebody that even their mom couldn't love properly? So, I did a lot of escaping through drugs. That was my escape. And then I met Paul and I found out that I really do matter. You know, I matter in real life, and I found out that I was really a nice person. And I really was *somebody*! I wasn't a nobody, like I had been made to believe all this time."

As her mental health condition began to improve, she developed other health problems. She started having trouble breathing, which was initially diagnosed as asthma but later, and more accurately, a pulmonary condition requiring open-heart surgery and a valve replacement. After that surgery in 2012, she felt she really wanted to do something different with her life.

Tonie studied and got her GED in 2013. And then she enrolled in the six-month program to train as a mental health and addiction peer specialist at Howie the Harp Advocacy Center in New York and began working there. She also decided to use her experience in the prison system and forensic medicine to do an internship at the Manhattan Psychiatric Center, which the Howie the Harp program funded.

And in 2015 she got her first paying job in mental health care. She was hired at CASES, the Center for Alternative Sentencing and Employment Services, a groundbreaking organization in New York that helps people with mental illness who have been recently arrested and those who have had mental health care in prison but need continued support after serving their sentences.

As a newSTART counselor for women at CASES, she attracted the attention of Dr. Elizabeth Ford at Columbia, who had previously been director of forensic psychiatry at Bellevue Hospital, and then reformed the mental health unit at Rikers Island (the same one that had been so useless when Tonie had been there much earlier). She was a pioneer in exploring the amazing potential of ambitious mental health care in jails and prisons. Dr. Ford was, during COVID, the medical director at CASES before joining the staff at Columbia University. (The two are close enough friends that when Tonie was recently hospitalized and needed to cancel a session with me for the book, Dr. Ford was the one who let me know.) Besides CASES, Tonie now also works as a crisis counselor for Miele's Respite in Jamaica, Queens, a crisis and counseling center that's part of Transitional Services for New York.

TONIE HAS CONTINUED to work with clients in person, on the phone, and through telehealth. She is in her New York office every other week. But she quietly decided to stop living in New York, and when there she stays at a friend's place. Her home is in another nearby state, close to longtime friends. She did this for her own safety. While she has been sober for nearly a decade, she continues to have issues with the men she falls for, who are sometimes violent and are sometimes still using. She needed to get away from that.

"I've had a lot of different men in my life," she said. "And I've let men take care of me." Men were even a challenge in recovery at twelve-step meetings. "I used to go to meetings, but the men look good to me," she said. "I found out men were also an addiction for me. And I just didn't want to do that. I slept with a lot of men when I was getting high. I didn't want to have to sleep with a lot of men. And when I put this last man out—and he wouldn't leave so I left—I made a decision. For the first time in my life, I'm single—and I'm celibate. I have had no sexual activity in my life for the last nine months. And I'm actually loving it. I'm actually loving the freedom of not having to coddle somebody else's emotions, because I really don't care about all of that."

She smiled broadly. "It sounds funny to hear me say that out loud."

Now that she is getting some perspective on sex, I was curious how she perceived it. Did she see herself as having a sexual compulsion? Or was it mostly transactional? Was the sex actually sex to her? Did it mean anything to her?

"No, not really. Not really," she said. "I have to question myself now. I don't really think that relationships meant that much to me. The people just don't mean that much to me. And I don't know if that is something that rolled over from all the abuse and trauma that I suffered as a child, molestation and stuff. But, yeah, people's feelings really don't mean a lot to me, because my feelings don't mean a lot to people."

Yet, the way she said this made it sound like she was trying to convince herself. Because Tonie seemed to be all about sharing feelings. During one of our last conversations, she started talking about her children—all of her children. The ones she remembers having and allowing family members to raise; the ones she barely remembers having, because she was high, and gave them up to social services or adoption.

"Look," she said, "I was a crack whore, okay? A crack ho' and I did a lot of things to survive. So now I'm clean, and I have these kids out there that don't know me. I have guilt over that. And I think that when I'm in pain, I'm *supposed* to be in pain."

She started crying. And then I heard a voice coming from the other room—this conversation was on Zoom—and a woman she called her "sister," but who is really a close family friend, interrupted the conversation so she could embrace and comfort her.

"You did the best you could," she kept telling Tonie as they hugged. And then the woman turned to me. "Let me tell you something about Miss Tonie," she said. "I met her when I was fifteen years old, and she was in her early twenties, and I was living with my child's father, and I did find out Tonie was getting high. But out of all the friends I had, whenever I need something, anything, even if it was money and she needed it to get high, she would give me the money right out of her pocket. No questions asked, didn't ask nothing in return. She has a very big heart, no matter what her situation is, and she's never gonna say no. Put it that way. She's never gonna say . . . I don't think she knows *how* to say no, especially when she sees someone that's in need."

Once Tonie calmed down and dried her cheeks, she grinned and continued.

"I'm very happy to say that my children are in my life," she said. "They love me. Like I was never gone."

How did you manage to reconnect with them?

"Facebook is amazing," she said. "There are the children that have been looking for me. My daughter who I call my 'mini-me' started a page called Tonie's Kids. And they all met on that page. And she doesn't allow anybody to say anything bad to her mother, not even her siblings. And if they think that they're gonna do it, she takes them off the page. Because she says that this is a page for us to bond and come together. It's not a page for bashing.

"I've given every one of them a platform for their feelings. Talk to me about how you feel. I suggest therapy. You know, I'm the one that damaged you, you're damaged. And it's because of me. And I want you to do what you need to do. When you're ready. If you want to sit down with me in therapy, that's fine. My son is thirty-two. And he and

I talk strongly about therapy, because he's really, really damaged—he's extremely damaged."

She sighed. "We talk all the time, text and things like that. I offered for him to sit with me in a session with my therapist, and that's something he's considering right now. But I have to be very present for him. If I tell him, 'Hey, I'm coming to New York this week, and I'll be there for this amount of time,' I *have to be there.* Because if I don't show up, he's still like that little boy whose mom has disappointed him yet again. And so, when I say something, I make sure that I do it. Because my children's lives are at stake. And I'm not going to rest until all of my children have treatment."

IN APRIL 2023, Tonie received word that one of her daughters was in critical condition in a hospital in South Carolina. She jumped on a plane to be with her, even though she had not set foot in South Carolina for over thirty years. When she arrived, her daughter was unconscious in the ICU, but during the week she was there at her bedside, she improved enough that Tonie felt it would be safe for her to return home. The experience of being in South Carolina was overwhelming, deeply triggering. And when she got back, she found herself having breakthrough symptoms—meaning they literally "broke through" what was normally her medical safety net of medication, talk therapy, and mindfulness—in a way she hadn't felt in years. There was psychosis, cycling between mania and depression. When I talked to her, she was upset, confused—and angry.

"I mean, I just want to know, is my mind cracking because of things that I remember from my past?" she asked. "Or is my mind cracking because of medication? With as much teaching as I do, I need to know, so I can educate others on mental health. I just thought that I was *exempt* from this now, I guess."

I told her I thought that was so interesting. Did you think, I asked, that the antipsychotic drugs just made the delusions go away? Or just that you didn't see them? Or that they weren't as bothersome? I've talked to other people involved with the book who also have different delusions. But since I don't have a psychotic illness myself, I'm always trying to figure out: Does it dampen the voices and allow you to ignore them? Or does it really make them go away? Or in your day-to-day life, does that not matter?

She paused for a second. "I thought that once I was well, mentally, that I was *well*," she said. "I didn't leave any room for the possibility of the voices returning, I didn't leave any space for becoming manic or depressed. I didn't leave any space for illness. I hope that I can get back to where I need to be before it's time for me to go to New York to go to work."

She did what she would have told a counseling client to do: she talked to her doctor, adjusted her meds and her sleeping, and went back to work. In fact, in early June, she spoke at a daylong symposium at Columbia, "Psychiatric Labels in the New York Pre-Trial Criminal Legal System: What Really Happens?" She was on a panel with the New York City Police Department's assistant commissioner of behavioral health and its triage sergeant, one of her bosses at CASES, and the medical director for crisis services for the state office of mental health.

A month later, she had returned to South Carolina for an extended visit. She looked healthier again, more centered. I asked her what was different.

"I'm with some of my kids," she said. One of her grandsons was spending the summer with her—the first time in his twelve years that she had ever spent any extended time with him. "He does so many things that remind me of my son, his father, who I wasn't always with," she said. "The way that he holds his head, the way he kisses me. I just feel so . . . honored that I can have those moments."

She was taking a little time away from counseling. "I just want to be close to my children," she said. "My mental health didn't go away. I have to remember I can't go twelve hours without sleep, I have to go to bed at night. I become delusional when I'm tired. I have to learn to accept that, take a step back when I need to, and not feel shame.

"I still talk to Paul every Tuesday; I'm not ever going to change that. I just really want to focus on some unfinished chapters that I need to go finish up. And that's my focus right now. I don't try to put too much on my plate. My appetite is not as big as it used to be. So, I'm only gonna put what I know I'm gonna digest on my plate."

She's thinking of buying a home so her children's children have a place of hers to visit. In the meantime, she is getting to know family from all stages of her life.

"This weekend," she said, "I got to hang out with my daughter who was in the hospital, who's the one my cousin raised, and my daughter whose father was in the military. They met for the first time. Their children met for the first time. My son's son met his aunts for the first time. And I had, I think . . . let me see, three, four, five, *six* of my grandchildren with me. It was a *lot* of emotions."

There were so many kids, from so many relationships, that she was trying to keep track of all the different things they called her. "Some of the North Carolina grandchildren call me MeeMa," she explained. "The ones from South Carolina call me Mom. One calls her mother Mom, so she calls me Ma.

"And my grandson, my son's son? Well, I'm his grandma," she beamed.

Chapter Five

Justin

In the fall of 2019, Justin Maffett was exactly where he wanted to be. In fact, given that he was only twenty-five, he might have been a couple of years ahead of himself. A tall, slim, handsome, engaging attorney from Tennessee—with an undergraduate degree from Dartmouth and a law degree from Columbia—he was a promising associate at the New York office of a top international law firm. But he had his eye on an eventual career in politics.

He had interned for a congressman in Washington, for the ACLU, for the Obama White House Office of Communications, and for MSNBC legal analyst and host Ari Melber. And while at MSNBC, he had become friendly with political and civil rights activist the Reverend Al Sharpton, who expressed an interest in mentoring him, calming his concerns that being Black and gay could be an impediment to being elected.

Over the next year, Justin had some struggles with typical rookie challenges of his first full-time job, and then the atypical challenges of the arrival of COVID and remote work: he was sworn into the New York Bar in May via Zoom in his Upper East Side apartment.

And then came the horrific killing of George Floyd in Minneapolis—which led him to actively join the New York protests. He even got arrested for breaking curfew during one of them.

In the heady excitement of the Black Lives Matter protests, everyone just assumed Justin was uniquely passionate about the cause. They had no idea—nor did Justin, really—that he was experiencing mania and was only months away from a complete psychotic break, during which he would become convinced he was an angel sent by God to save the country from racism, Russia, and China.

He also had no idea just how quickly someone who is ill and delusional, but still very resourceful and ambitious, can tear down so much of what it took a lifetime to carefully create. In just two months, he found himself in psychiatric hospitals three times. He not only lost his job but was charged criminally by one of his former bosses. He ran up tens of thousands of dollars in credit card debt. He had confrontations with security at the FBI, the CIA, the White House, and the vice president's house. And he went off on family and friends about anything they had ever done that bothered him.

"I thought I was lighting the world on fire," Justin told me, "when all I was doing was burning bridges."

But he considers himself lucky: he was properly diagnosed with bipolar disorder in a matter of weeks, when for some people it takes months or even years to receive, and then accept, the stunning verdict of chronic illness. And this was accomplished during an unusually mentally challenging period in the country—including the 2020 election and the January 6 attack on the Capitol. He was also fortunate his disorder responded well to medication and talk therapy.

He is anxious to share his story not only because he feels it will help others but because he believes strongly that people with mental illnesses should be able to share their medical challenges without shame like everyone else with every other disease.

"Putting what it means to be manic into words is very difficult," Justin said. "There's this rush of emotions, these feelings of powerfulness and immunity, where you are on top of the world and nobody can stop you. Just me against the world. It's a high you can't buy, almost pure adrenaline. I felt like I was a character in a movie. Your imagination takes hold of you, and it becomes your reality. I was convinced I was in the middle of a geopolitical conflict and the CIA was involved and my law firm was complicit and, well, it makes for a fascinating tale—unless it actually happens to *you*. I said a lot of hurtful things during a state of psychosis that you really can't take back."

But he has had the courage not only to try but to keep trying.

JUSTIN MAFFETT GREW UP an only child in a succession of college towns. His father was a university fundraiser—first at Yale, then at the University of Maryland, and finally in Nashville at Cumberland University and Meharry Medical College—and his mother was a nurse. The family was active in the Baptist church. He was bright, excelled in private school, and went to sleepaway camp in the summer. His only significant childhood health issue was asthma.

Justin came out at age fifteen, during his sophomore year in high school, but not on purpose. He accidentally left pornography on the computer the family shared at home; his father found it and woke him up in the middle of the night to confront him, and then insisted he tell his mother. He remembered the time as being tense, and his mother being more upset than his father.

But he also remembered something much bigger happening later that same year: his father lost his fundraising job, and over the next years, while he did consulting work, his mother became the family's main breadwinner. There was financial stress, although Justin was able to get scholarships for private school and then Dartmouth.

Justin did well in college but sought help in his junior year for what turned out to be ADHD. He got therapy and was prescribed the stimulant medication dextroamphetamine/amphetamine (Adderall), which he took for the rest of college. At Columbia Law School, he continued talk therapy and was switched to the nonstimulant ADHD medicine atomoxetine (Strattera). He smoked pot and drank, rarely to excess. He sometimes wondered if he might have some mood instability, but it was never diagnosed or treated. He was sexually active but had yet to have a long-term relationship. His energy went into school and internships.

As an undergrad he spent a summer in the D.C. office of his congressman in Tennessee, Jim Cooper, then a summer in the D.C. office of the ACLU. The summer before law school he interned in the White House Office of Communications during the last months of the Obama administration. He had a challenging time that summer, finding himself anxious, depressed, and often tearful in the aftermath of the mass shooting at Pulse, a gay nightclub in Orlando. "In the White House Office of Communications, we had a front row seat to all this tragedy," he recalled. "I was starting to break down." But he was able to work through it, finish his internship, and go to law school. He saw the mood changes as being justified by external events.

During his second and third years in law school, he was also working at MSNBC in New York as an intern for Ari Melber's daily show, and then as a legal news writer for Melber's appearances as legal correspondent for NBC News. That's where he met Rev. Al

Sharpton, who in addition to his weekend news show and other appearances on MSNBC, did a radio show in the same building at Rockefeller Center and invited Justin to visit him there on Fridays, which he began doing regularly. They talked about politics, and Justin shared that while he wanted to work for a law firm for a few years, his dream was to run for Congress in New York, like Representative Hakeem Jeffries (who he had also met to discuss his political future). He and Sharpton had long, frank discussions almost every Friday. Justin was concerned that being Black and comfortably out could hurt his chances of one day becoming a congressman; Sharpton assured him times had changed, and it wouldn't hurt his chances any more than it had prevented him from becoming a lawyer.

Justin spent his last law school summer as an associate at the New York office of Debevoise & Plimpton, an international law firm that prided itself on its diversity, and when he graduated, they offered him a full-time job. He was especially pleased that they didn't ask him to tone down his stylish way of dressing for work. On his first day, he had a cell phone picture taken of him posing in front of the firm's logo in a white shirt, slim black pants, loafers, and no socks. When he posted it on his LinkedIn page, he wrote, "Part of me still struggles to believe it's all real, especially when you remember how few of us black/LGBT folk are in corporate law at elite NYC law firms, even in 2019." His substantial salary allowed him to rent a spacious apartment at Eighty-fifth and York, with high ceilings and big windows.

The work was challenging, and sometimes he felt overwhelmed. In November 2019, after one of his mentors at the firm was hard on him, he experienced what he later realized was an anxiety attack—fear, panic, pain in his chest and stomach. He had felt this a couple of times in college and law school and was prescribed medication he could take just when he was symptomatic, which quickly helped. (He was prescribed the benzodiazepine lorazepam [Ativan], which has many different uses in mental health care, but is usually preferred for short-term use, "as needed," because overuse can lead to addiction.) He continued to feel some pressure at work, but it seemed normal for a first-year associate.

In March 2020, like everyone else in New York, Justin started working from home because of COVID. He found living alone very isolating, and to cope, what had been his weekend use of alcohol and pot began encroaching on his work hours. He rarely left home for the next several months, until the Black Lives Matter protests began in New York in June. Then he headed to the streets.

He took a leadership role in the protests, gave impassioned speeches, and was arrested once for breaking curfew for a protest. He became cochair of the Racial Justice Working Group of the Four Freedoms Democratic Club on the Upper East Side, and not only wrote stories about racial equity but was written about. Legal reporters noted with interest and appreciation how his big firm supported his increasing social activism.

The work was invigorating and heady, and it made Justin think harder about running for public office. While some suggested he run for the state legislature, Justin was more interested in the U.S. House of Representatives. His mentors at the law firm were politically connected. They seemed supportive when he floated the idea that he might cut back on his banking law practice to explore a midterm run in 2022. He started talking to people who might help him raise money. To look the part, he decided he needed a nice car. On October 29, he ordered a Tesla Model 3 for $41,790.

As he got more excited about running for office that fall, he also started experiencing what he later realized was mania—his thoughts were racing in a way that at first seemed exciting, and then became uncontrollable, overwhelming. And then he starting hearing thoughts that he believed were not entirely his own, voices telling him he was an angel of God.

The feeling was not entirely unfamiliar.

Once, a year earlier, when he was at his peak of frenzy studying for the bar exam—and overusing alcohol and his vape pen—he had felt this way. It was during a lost weekend that he had spent lying on the hardwood floor of his Upper East Side apartment, arms extended like he was on a cross, listening to a voice say, "You are special, you are an angel of God." On the first day he received the news that he was an angel; on the second he had been told what that meant: "something like a commission into an army." And the third day he had been informed that his mission was all wrapped up in his political ambitions, and "by going into politics, I could affect the change that I thought God wanted to see." He had finally left his apartment late Sunday afternoon, still with a heightened feeling of religiosity, and had walked to Fifth Avenue, where he entered the first church he could find and prayed. Then he saw a Peter Pan bus drive by, which made him think of Saint Peter, leading him to jump in a cab and follow the bus to St. Patrick's Basilica, almost seventy blocks away. He went in looking for priests to speak to, but all the services were over, so he went to another church. Finally, he got into a discussion with a homeless man named Charlie, who he talked to about accepting Christ.

Afterward, he returned home and started feeling more normal. The next day he called his psychiatrist—who, up to this point, was mostly treating him for ADHD and occasional anxiety—and told him something was wrong. But since the symptoms had stopped, the psychiatrist had felt the episode sounded like a temporary reaction to the bar exam pressures.

But in December 2020, after nine months of living alone and working from home because of COVID, the symptoms he thought were an aberration returned, and again he was thinking about being an angel of God on a mission. He had all but stopped eating and lost twenty pounds off his already slim frame. He found himself talking more rapidly, sometimes nonstop, and not always seeming coherent and intelligible to others. But he believed he could still fake normalcy when necessary.

He had told a politically connected friend, who was also a modern art collector, that he was exploring his political options and might want to finish decorating his big empty apartment for media interviews. In December, the friend offered to loan him some art he had bought but wasn't currently displaying.

Justin chose one piece that appealed to him, a painting by David Paul Kay titled *Scream,* an imposing, four-by-three-foot, black-and-white, abstract face in full shriek. "I was immediately struck by it," he recalled. "It captured my feelings of psychological torment and confusion, which I had been feeling for a while and nobody else could imagine. While I didn't know I was manic, I was aware that *something* was happening to me, a thrilling storm of mind-splitting ideas that bent my sense of reality."

His friend had the painting wrapped for safe transport, and Justin brought it home. Until he could get it framed, he leaned it, still wrapped, against the wall in his living room.

Not long after, Justin called Ari Melber's show to insist they put him on to talk about racism; they stopped returning his calls. Al Sharpton invited him to join him and his daughter at his Harlem office as they helped feed the homeless for the holidays. But when Justin arrived, it was clear something about him wasn't right. He was talking too fast, perspiring, and had a dazed look in his eye; he was making proclamations, saying he was running for president. As a minister, Sharpton had seen behavior like this before, but he didn't know if it was the result of drugs or mental illness. And then they never heard from him again.

By Christmas 2020, Justin had all but lost complete control of his thoughts. It is a process that is challenging to describe or document, but Justin shared my interest in trying to make these feelings and symptoms more understandable. So he gave us hospital bills, criminal complaints, cease and desist letters, emails, texts, and receipts, detailing all kinds of personal and professional mayhem. They offer a powerful psychiatric travelogue of how quickly waves of manic psychosis can explode and implode your life.

On the day before Christmas, Justin decided to unwrap the *Scream* painting so he could think about what kind of frame he wanted for it. He found himself staring at the contorted *Scream* face, unable to look away. He became convinced that his friend had commissioned the painting *just for him,* because he knew it captured the unique feelings inside his head.

Justin also understood that the painting was worth a lot of money, at least $25,000, and this realization triggered in him "a moment of religious self-righteousness, of trying to reject materialism.

"I was thinking, 'What the fuck is my life, how did I go from being some kid in Nashville to being on the cusp of running for office on the Upper East Side, driving a Tesla, and now I have a $25,000 painting in my apartment?'"

Suddenly, the voice in his head told him to grab something sharp. He found a pair of scissors and slashed the canvas, from the top of one eye across to the bottom of the mouth. Then he did it again from the other eye.

Just an hour or two later, the voices told Justin he needed to take a train to Washington and get a job at the White House. So he called the concierge service for his credit card, arranged for an Amtrak ticket, and took the next train to D.C. During the ride, he sent several disjointed texts from the train, including one to Sharpton floating the idea that maybe the reverend could help him be named a U.S. ambassador.

Then Justin got into an argument with the man sitting in the seat ahead of him, who he thought was talking too loud on his cell phone. When Justin wouldn't stop harassing the man, a conductor was called. Justin was accused of being "crazy" and they arranged for him to be escorted off the train at the next stop, which was Philadelphia.

Justin took a cab to the airport and then a shuttle bus to the car rental lot. By then it was after 7:00 P.M., and it was raining. Avis was out of cars, so he walked in the rain to the Hertz building and rented one of their most expensive cars, a Volvo XC 90, at a rate of $370 a day.

He drove in the rain to Washington. When he arrived at the White House, he was, of course, refused admission but was kindly told it was because he didn't have an appointment. The voices then told him, "Your mission isn't the White House anyway. You need to be at the CIA." So he drove there. CIA Security was less friendly—they surrounded his car and told him to turn around and not return.

He then called one of his bosses from the law firm and asked if he would help him find a place to stay in D.C. for Christmas. When the partner seemed confused and put off, Justin got it in his head that the people at his firm had turned on him. He decided to drive back to New York, and as he did, he became more and more incensed. He stopped in Philadelphia, tried to check into the Four Seasons, but was asked to leave, and then checked into the Downtown Sheraton to shower and get cleaned up. He also started emailing his mentors at the law office—copying the messages to the firm's senior partners. His emails accused them of coming up short in diversity and racial equity, as well as conspiring to help him get elected only so he would be able to get their children jobs. He claimed he would have one of his mentors arrested for bribing him as a potential candidate.

After being at the hotel for only an hour, he got back in the rental car and drove toward New York. But in his manic state, he failed to pay attention to the gas indicator and ran out of gas on the New Jersey Turnpike. Police came and the car was towed, but Justin just asked them to take him to the closest train station. He needed to get back to New York right away. He was convinced the FBI and local police were about to arrest his mentor for attempting to bribe him, and he needed to be there.

In New York, he called the firm's car service, which, even though it was Christmas Day, was immediately dispatched to pick him up. And when he asked to be taken to the Brooklyn home of one of the firm's partners, the service knew the address and figured there was a valid reason.

When Justin got there, he was stunned: "I didn't see any cop cars, no FBI vehicles. I didn't see any prosecutors. I was really confused," he explained. "I felt I had been very clear in my directions and, as an angel of the Lord, had commanded them to arrest this man."

Finally, Justin walked up to the brownstone and stepped into the vestibule because the doors were unlocked. He rang the bell, and when nobody answered, he picked up a fire extinguisher and went out to his boss's Tesla Model S. He proceeded to bang on the car windows with the fire extinguisher, marking them up, and then he took a key out of his pocket and scraped it along the side of the car.

He then got back into the company car and had the driver take him to a Thai restaurant. He told the waitress he was feeling very high, and at the end of the meal he tipped her $100. She asked if he wanted more water, and he asked for a glass of wine. And when it arrived, he got it into his head that he had changed the water into wine. Then he went home where, in his anger, he trashed his apartment.

The next day he took a cab to Midtown but didn't bring his wallet. When the cabbie realized he couldn't pay, he called the police and drove Justin to the closest precinct. There Justin was told he could either pay or be arrested. According to the police report, Justin said, "Go ahead then, arrest me!" They did. He was taken to a holding cell where he was "jumping up and down" and "verbalizing suicidal ideation." So, police transferred him to the emergency department at Bellevue Hospital.

"I was walking through the Bellevue ER in full chains, shackles, as I was under arrest," he recalled. "There was so much embarrassment and shame. Even while psychotic, I recognized what I was being put through, even though I wasn't a threat to anyone." He was still talking nonstop about his "friends in high places"—including President Obama and other "government people"—and the "signs" he was noticing "that people are against me."

He did make one comment that had some possible medical logic—he wondered if the marijuana he had been smoking could have been "spiked" with something. The issue of "laced weed" was a real one, with both law enforcement and marijuana advocates worried about cocaine, PCP, or even fentanyl being mixed with cannabis. If Justin's symptoms had turned out to be temporary, that could be a possible explanation for his psychosis.

Either way, the symptoms still needed to be treated. He was given an injection of antipsychotic medicine, which sedated him.

He was treated at Bellevue for three days. During that time, the hospital got in touch with his employers, who confirmed that they were very concerned about his recent behavior. The doctors at Bellevue were finally able to convince him that he met criteria for a psychotic episode (he told them he preferred the term "mental break") but they weren't clear why it had happened or if it would happen again. His tox screens turned out to be negative for anything that could have "spiked" his marijuana.

On New Year's Eve at 12:56 P.M., Justin was discharged from the hospital. His diagnosis was a psychotic episode; he was sent home with prescriptions for olanzapine (Zyprexa), an antipsychotic, and lorazepam, the same benzodiazepine sedative he'd been prescribed "as needed" the year before. However, according to his charts, he told the doctors he felt his case had been mismanaged and he really didn't need medication.

He left with his mother, who had driven up from his parents' home in Richmond, Virginia. As soon as they were outside the front door of the hospital, the police came and arrested Justin. As his mother stood there perplexed, he was told there was a warrant out for his arrest.

While he was in the hospital, his firm had sent him a registered letter informing him he had been fired, he had to cease and desist from all contact with anyone at his law firm, and that his behavior had "crossed the line into criminal conduct" and had "caused members of the firm community and their families to fear for their safety." His mentor had also filed a criminal complaint against him: eleven charges including aggravated harassment, burglary and attempted burglary, criminal mischief with intent to damage, and disorderly conduct. As evidence, they offered video from the exterior camera of his mentor's next-door neighbor, which had captured the whole incident. He spent that night in jail in Brooklyn and the next day was released.

For the next few days, Justin proceeded as if this had been an isolated incident. He still wasn't completely himself, but he felt well enough that his mother went back home, and he attempted to begin repairing his life. He had a friend from home, who was in the military, as well as one of his closest colleagues from the BLM protests write letters of recommendation and explanation for him.

But his mind soon started revving up again. During the afternoon of January 6, he called the concierge at his credit card company again to make reservations to return to Washington. He had no idea what had been unfolding there that day. The concierge said, "Don't you know what's going on? People have stormed the Capitol!" He wasn't all that surprised.

"To a manic person," he explained, "everything is that dramatic and it can often sound like the world is ending. It only confirmed my deep suspicion of a grand conspiracy. I mean, what an incredible event to happen while you're manic."

He had the concierge book him a rental car, he packed a bag, and, before leaving his apartment later that day, he decided he needed to bring the slashed *Scream* painting with him.

"It was like a relic of some sort," he recalled. "I thought it spoke to some deeper conspiracy."

He drove down to D.C. in the middle of the night. He parked at the Capitol Hilton at 8:46 A.M., and then started walking around the Capitol area, while they were locking down after the attack. Dressed in jeans and a hoodie, he met and chatted with some militia members who had been involved in the events the day before. Then he called his godfather, who lived in town, to see if he might be able to stay with him that night.

Probably the only really lucky thing about Justin's entire experience was that his godfather was someone who could really help him—Arthur Evans, PhD, the chief executive officer of the American Psychological Association and the former Commissioner for Behavioral Health for the City of Philadelphia. When Justin was born, Evans attended the same church as his parents in Connecticut, and the families stayed in touch. (Arthur is also a longtime public health colleague of mine, which is how I met Justin.)

When Justin called to see if he could stay, Arthur's wife thought he didn't sound right. This was also during the height of COVID, before anyone had been vaccinated, so she suggested he stay at a hotel, and Arthur would come visit him. He stayed at the Hilton one night, but because he heard that Proud Boys were staying there, he moved across Sixteenth Street, with the painting, to the St. Regis.

Over those two days, he was overpaying taxis to take him around the D.C. area, trying to gain entry to the White House and FBI headquarters again—and this time he was turned away much more brusquely. He also went to the CIA headquarters and the vice president's house, all in an effort to tell officials what he knew about the Capitol attack and warn them about a coming threat to the United States from China. While some of the security personnel he encountered seemed to understand he was manic, he was also able to convince them that he wasn't a threat. The fact that nobody arrested him on January 7—one of the scariest days in the history of the U.S. Capitol—is a testimony to how, even floridly psychotic, he still was able to summon his ability to talk and think like a lawyer.

At the end of the day, he returned to the St. Regis, where he found himself pacing so much—not uncommon during mania—that he asked for a bigger room with more walking space. He and the *Scream* painting were moved to a $700-a-night suite, which overlooked the

"Black Lives Matter" mural painted in yellow letters fifty feet tall on Sixteenth Street. He ordered room service, twice, watched MSNBC, and finally connected with his godfather, who came over.

"I'm talking with him, and he's clearly experiencing psychosis," Arthur told me. "He's not making a lot of sense. He said he was in town to get a job, was having conversations with people at the White House. And, on the surface, he's holding it together. I knew he did an internship at the White House, so it's just credible enough that you can say, 'Okay, well, maybe that's true.' But as the night went on, what he was saying just wasn't adding up. He said he was there because he wanted to protect people, like he was on some kind of mission.

"And then at some point, I said to him, 'Justin, you might be having some problems. It might be good for you to see someone.' And he got very angry with me."

Arthur was especially concerned because of what was happening in Washington at that time. "A lot of his delusion centered around law enforcement, which really kind of scared me," he said, "because here's a young Black man who clearly is having mental health challenges, going up talking to law enforcement." After two hours of listening to Justin manically go on, Arthur left at 1:00 A.M.—he didn't think Justin was a danger to himself—and said he'd be back in the morning. When he returned, he convinced Justin to go with him to the emergency department of nearby Sibley Memorial Hospital.

But they didn't have a room for him. So Arthur ended up sitting there with him in the emergency department for the next twenty-four hours, both of them masked to prevent COVID, and each getting maybe an hour or two of sleep. He kept Justin's parents apprised of what was going on.

The next morning, Justin agreed to go by ambulance to MedStar

Washington Hospital, about thirty minutes away, where they had a bed in the psychiatry unit for him. Arthur was able to monitor his care and speak to his psychiatrist; Justin also called him periodically from one of the two phones in the middle of the unit's main hallway. While he improved at MedStar, Justin was still not completely convinced that what he was experiencing was a disease process from a mental illness—it still felt situational to him, and certainly the country was in an unprecedented situation. He was particularly upset that staff members seemed not to believe anything he said.

"There was a nurse-tech at MedStar who refused to believe I was a lawyer," he recalled. "She literally said, 'A lawyer wouldn't act this way.' I jumped on the ground and started flailing around and making strange noises, and asked, 'What does a lawyer look like or sound like?' Finally, I saw her sitting at one of the computers, and I asked her to google my name. She said she couldn't because of HIPAA." (HIPAA, the Health Insurance Portability and Accountability Act of 1996, includes patient confidentiality rules that are important but are often invoked too broadly; they do not preclude a patient from sharing his own information.)

"I said, 'Fuck HIPAA. I'm giving you permission,'" he recalled. "This is post–George Floyd protests, my name is *very* google-able. The first hit was a story about charges being dropped against me in New York, and me working toward getting them dropped for others. She went silent."

Justin was discharged from MedStar after ten days. His condition was better, but his discharge summary shows he declined to even have a discharge plan on departing—so no mental health care plan, no medical plan. And he admitted he was "not connected to services" and was "looking for a therapist." He didn't even tell the hospital where to send his records.

While this is far from ideal, and many experts would say it isn't medically safe, it happens every day. Also, Justin insisted upon it—and ultimately, the patient has the right to depart without a plan.

In retrospect, Arthur bemoaned that this happened and wished he had been there when Justin was released. While he didn't physically see Justin when he was discharged, and can't say for sure he wasn't well enough to be released, "Not having an immediate connection to care is *always* a problem for people, especially if they're having a first psychotic episode. I've heard experts say that some scary number like ninety percent of people in Justin's situation would be sent home without a treatment plan that they could begin the very next day."

When Arthur was Philadelphia's behavioral health commissioner, he often talked to hospital administrators about this issue. "It's pretty clear that the longer the time between discharge and the first outpatient appointment, the more likely people are to relapse," he said. "Hospitals told us they couldn't do anything about this. So, we started offering financial incentives: we would give them a performance payment if they were able to increase what we call 'connection to care rates,' which would reduce relapses among their discharged patients. And since this could add up to really large payments, these same providers, all of a sudden, got very creative. This is an issue of *will*. It's not rocket science."

JUSTIN TOOK A train back to New York, unaccompanied. Arthur had arranged for a caregiver in New York to connect with Justin, but it didn't happen quickly enough. Within a day, Justin was manic again. He went on a shopping spree and spent thousands of dollars on clothes. He checked into the Park Lane Hotel on Central Park South—even though he had an apartment three subway stops away—because he thought "the end of the world was near" and it was a better place to "bunker." He called Arthur, letting him know, "I have access to the nuclear codes."

Arthur convinced him to go back to his apartment, and then he called New York authorities and informed them that Justin was in a mental health crisis. An emergency response team came to his apartment and convinced him to go with them to nearby Metropolitan Hospital. In the emergency department, Justin tested positive for COVID—the conspiratorial causes of which Justin explained in detail to anyone who would listen. So, he had to be treated in isolation for fourteen days before coming to the psychiatric unit. But he was started immediately on the medication for a diagnosis of bipolar I, the more serious of the two bipolar diagnoses. The initial treatment of choice is lithium combined with something else to relieve other symptoms. In Justin's case he was started on lithium and gabapentin (Neurontin), an anti-seizure medication that is also effective in treating extreme restlessness and impulsivity.

His mother rushed up from Virginia; she visited him every day and spent much of the rest of the time cleaning up his apartment, which he had trashed, and doing his laundry. It was not easy for her to be around him, because he was still psychotic and part of his ranting turned to her and all the ways she had failed him as a mother. He recalled being forcibly medicated and placed in four-point restraints (wrists and ankles attached to the bed) and six-point restraints (shoulders also attached), left in them for longer than he thought could possibly be necessary.

"I was clawing at my restraints, trying to bite them off," he recalled. "I asked them to take them off me. They just stood there and tried to console me. I shit in a bed pan and peed into one of those containers while fully restrained. It was not only embarrassing but traumatizing. Any time I think about being restrained by all four limbs, I start to cry, even if I'm by myself. It's so scary."

By the time he was cleared of COVID and able to be treated in the inpatient psychiatry unit, his symptoms had improved somewhat. But he was still delusional and hostile enough—primarily angry at not being fully believed—that the antipsychotic medication haloperidol (Haldol) was added. The combination of the lithium and haloperidol soon made an impact.

"It's hard to explain what that's like because I don't really remember everything," he told me. "The deeply psychotic moments are kind of like, when you go under anesthesia, you remember them giving you the medicine and counting down but you don't really remember the experience of actually falling asleep. But there comes a point when you do start remembering. It's not like in the movies where one day you start asking, 'Where have I been?' and the nurses tell you, 'Oh, he's back, y'all.' It's more gradual. And I think they could tell because I started asking more questions."

Part of his reconnection to reality was finally being able to piece together his multiple hospitalizations over such a short period, combined with what his doctors were telling him and what Arthur was assuring him, that he had bipolar disorder, and he needed to accept and treat it, every day. The politics of the day, no matter how extreme, were not the main reason he had blown up so much of his professional and personal life.

On February 16, 2021, Justin was discharged from the hospital in his mother's care. She drove him back to their family home in Virginia, and he began a new life with a chronic illness—a treatable illness, but one that he realized was not going to go away. He also began the long process of addressing all the charges and paying all the bills he had run up during three months of psychosis. He wondered, sometimes, how much worse it would have gone for him had his godfather not been the head of the American Psychological Association.

His godfather wonders the same thing. "Mental health systems are so overly complicated and opaque, I have no idea how the average person can navigate them," he told me. "With as much as I know, it was still very difficult for me to help Justin get the care he needed. The only way I could do it was to call in favors from people. And these are big city systems where they at least have resources. It's not like small or rural communities where there's very little access. I was also struck by how every city is so different—and even sections of cities were different—in how they handle mental health crises. If you have a heart attack, you call 911, they give you CPR, and you are taken to an emergency department. If you have a mental health emergency, it's often unclear which crisis service takes you to which hospital, and afterward where you're supposed to get continuing care. There are rarely standard pathways for help. It's a huge problem."

One of the many things Justin had to do to move on from his acute illness was to deal with the *Scream* painting. He took it to an art restorer, hoping that neither the friend who loaned it nor the artist would ever find out he had slashed it. The restorer said it could be fixed for $2,500. What he didn't mention was that he would actually need the artist to do some repainting. Justin only found out about this later, when the artist was interviewed by a journalist doing a story on art restoration. He was pleasantly surprised to learn that the artist completely understood Justin had been ill when he damaged the work. The painter admitted that he had been struggling with mental illness himself when he created the painting. He felt that the saga of the repair "added a new layer of emotional symbolism and meta-history" to the work.

I MET JUSTIN about a year after he came home. By then, he had been able to take care of all of his legal situations: he ended up pleading out to "disorderly conduct," which in New York is not a criminal offense, while all the other charges were dropped. And his treatment with medication and psychotherapy had been successful. He remained on lithium—which can be a bit of a challenge to take because it works best in a narrow therapeutic range, so patients need to be blood tested periodically. But when it works, being a "lithium responder" is a good thing for those with bipolar disorder. And he has taken the lithium every day without fail since being discharged from the hospital.

His psychiatrist added another medication, aripiprazole (Abilify), an antipsychotic that is also widely used as a mood stabilizer for bipolar disorder and unipolar depression. He began taking the aripiprazole every day. But then, in consultation with his psychiatrist, he switched to taking it only when he felt he needed it. (Unlike some mental health medicines, which need time to start working, antipsychotics usually make a more immediate impact.) Recently, he hasn't felt he needed it at all—but he has the pills if that changes.

"I definitely take it when I've had a weird dream or my mind starts to think faster," he said. "When I have felt my brain revving up, I will take the antipsychotic just to make sure that I don't veer into a manic episode."

I asked if he could better explain why he doesn't take a medication daily that he knows works—not to criticize him in any way, but because I know that many people do this in consultation with their psychiatrists. I know I have. We experiment. We also give ourselves what pharmacologists call "drug holidays"—often without talking to our doctors about it. It's especially true for drugs like antipsychotics, which can be sedating and dull the senses.

"There's just something about being put on an antipsychotic every single day that makes me feel a certain type of way," he said. "I'm not actively psychotic. So, why do I need to be on an antipsychotic every single day?"

So, I asked, are you making a medical decision for a more psychological reason?

"I wouldn't say psychological. I think I mean it more *philosophically,*" he said. "Also, ever since I was a kid, I've gone through waves of inspiration and creativity. Post-diagnosis, I've been a little more critical of those waves—are they inspiration because I'm a creative type, or is this the beginning of a manic episode? So, I just want to feel a little more personally in control of that. Does that make sense?"

It does, especially since far too many patients let those kinds of thoughts lead them to stop taking all their meds, sometimes secretly, and often with disastrous consequences. Justin takes his lithium "religiously."

WHEN I MET Justin, he was still struggling with some of the consequences of his six weeks of intense illness and remained unsure if he should reach out to all those he had hurt, criticized, or vandalized, to let them know he had been ill. But he was thinking about the future, trying to decide if he should go back to corporate law or try something else. Much to his pleasant surprise, he got another job as a corporate attorney in the Washington office of another international firm for an even higher salary than his previous job. It allowed him to pay off all his credit card debts, but he didn't love the work, which was even more technical than his previous job. After five months, he started feeling depressed and, unclear if this was just a return of his symptoms or a response to the work, he requested a medical leave.

During the interview process for the job, Justin had explained that the gap in his employment record was because "I had been hospitalized for health issues" without explaining what they were. And nobody asked. Now, he told the head of his group about his bipolar diagnosis, and the firm was accommodating and supportive. During his leave, Justin decided he needed to get away from everything, so he packed a bag (including his medication) and backpacked through eight countries in Europe and South America. After three months on disability, he decided he could not go back, left the firm, and started thinking about an entirely new direction for his life.

He told me he had completely given up on his political aspirations, in part because he believed his mental health history would be used against him. I told him I hoped he was wrong about his illness being a reason he couldn't seek public office—or any career he wanted. I asked him if he was going to reach out to any of his mentors and explain what had really happened.

When he said he wasn't ready to, I asked if it would be okay if I reached out on his behalf to Rev. Al Sharpton, who knows my family. Justin said that would be fine.

Sharpton was pleased to hear that Justin was doing well, and he completely understood—once I explained it to him—that Justin had been in the throes of a manic-psychotic episode. I asked if he was open to Justin reaching out and reconnecting.

"Sure," he said. "I think that mental health is a major problem in this country, and probably disproportionately in our community. I'm glad he's telling his story, and I think it could give people courage to step up in our community. Justin had promise. He had what we call 'the package': he was smart, he had some charisma, and some hunger and determination. I'm always in search of young people who *get it.* He was very bright and very ambitious, and mostly what we had been talking about was how people would receive his sexuality if he ran for office."

Sharpton had told him then that he shouldn't worry about being "out" when considering a run for Congress. And he felt the same way about mental health.

"Mental illness is not something that ought to be looked down on," he said. "It's something that we ought to deal with like we deal with any other illness."

JUSTIN WAS INTRIGUED to learn that Sharpton was open to reconciliation and even political mentorship. But he felt strongly that his mental health crisis had brought him perspective he might never have otherwise had about where his talent and ambition should be focused.

"I was able to get back to work pretty fast," he explained. "But in terms of really internalizing and coming to terms with my diagnosis, and what that meant for my life, and my professional aspirations, I don't think I had fully grappled with that yet. And it took time to see that if I really wanted more balance in my life, if I really wanted to incorporate my diagnosis into my day-to-day, I needed to pursue other ventures than corporate law.

"For me, a more authentic path was one that was more creative and had more flexibility. If you read about the kind of career paths that people with bipolar disorder pursue or need, they need that flexibility. By going on a kind of world tour, I pushed myself to reengage with people and reengage with the world. And it kind of jump-started my personality, which I felt I had lost after being hospitalized for so long, and having, literally, kind of lost my mind and my senses. And so, after traveling to all these countries, and backpacking and hanging out in airport lounges and talking to business people, I decided to change direction."

Always interested in fashion and business as well as law, and eager to explore living abroad, Justin started looking at graduate school programs in Paris that might combine his skills. He also explored, "as an experiment to push and challenge myself," starting a men's fashion company that could produce suits especially for travelers, using sustainable and alternative fabrics. He even put up a website for the company, which he named Dunnock, after a sparrow-like European bird, migrating between endangered habitats, which "unaware of its short time on earth . . . nevertheless naturally knows to travel to some of the most beautiful areas of the world to pass its precious time."

He ultimately decided business school made more sense for him right now than entrepreneurship, and in the late summer of 2023, with his thirtieth birthday looming, he began a five-year PhD program in Law and Regulation at HEC Paris, one of the world's best business schools. He studies the relationships between city and regional governments and how they can interact on international relations and foreign policy issues.

He has also developed a relationship with the Office of Global Partnerships at the U.S. State Department, where he began as a volunteer subnational diplomacy legislation advisor. Justin hopes this can turn into something more permanent at the State Department while he finishes his degree.

"A part of me is beginning to think it might be safe to revisit my aspirations of government service and politics," he said. "Maybe my story does come kind of full circle after all."

Chapter Six

Ashley

When I met Ashley Dunlop, she was a health-care aide for elderly patients in the Nashville area. She was in her midthirties, moonfaced with a hopeful smile and a slight drawl. She and her husband, Drew, who is more than twenty years her elder, had been married for just under three years. They were starting to think about children. But there were challenges.

"We went to Walmart and got a pair of little baby slippers that were little gray koalas," she told me. "And then Drew hung them on the wall."

Why?

"He said, 'The next time you want to *use,* look at those baby slippers and remember that we're trying to have a family. That's what we're trying to do. And every time you use, you put that off a little more.'"

She paused for a second.

"And I didn't feel guilty when I looked at the slippers and then I used," she admitted. "But it was a reminder that I do have a goal in life, I do want to be a mother."

I asked how long ago he put them up. She had told me just how fragile her recovery from crack cocaine use has been, how often she has relapsed, and how, with the support of her husband and her integrated care team at Vanderbilt, she hopefully begins again.

"They've been up for a year," she explained. "I mean, he just wanted to put a visual reminder, 'That's not the choice that you need to make,' without actually *saying* that. He never once told me, 'You can't do this or I'll leave you, or I'll kick you out.' He allowed me to be sick. But he was still there for me. He didn't wildly enable me. But he was there, he supported me. He would hold me when I walked in from three days of being up all night and day, running and hustling in the streets. I would just collapse into the bed, and he would hold me. I would sob, I would cry, I didn't want to be doing it. But he would still support me."

Does she share about this in her twelve-step meetings?

"Nobody understands that," she said. "They think it's straight enabling. And they don't understand that kind of love. They do not."

If we want to truly help people with mental illnesses and addictions, we need to better understand that kind of love.

ASHLEY FIRST STARTED having auditory hallucinations as a teenager in a small suburb of Nashville, where the largest employer was a company that made water heaters. She experienced what she called "radio talking," steady muffled voices always commenting, as well as "game show style" voices, repeatedly calling out her name as if she was being introduced as a contestant, but also criticizing her. They initially repeated things she had actually heard others say to her, or about her, that had stung when she was in junior high.

"It's like they began as feelings," she explained, "and later on turned into voices." She didn't realize what they were until many years later.

Ashley drank and smoked pot as a teenager as a way of self-medicating against the voices and feelings of depression and agitation. She acted out sexually, primarily with older men.

"Let me see how to word this," she said. "I see now how I thought that I had control in the realm of sex and sexual intercourse. I was sleeping with men who were in their thirties and forties, and I felt like I was the one in control. In fact, the only thing I had control of in my life at that point was the ability to attract men and get what I wanted out of them. Not money necessarily, but just control."

She doesn't recall her parents being sympathetic. She told me they thought she was "faking" her symptoms as some kind of "pity card to get people to feel sorry for me."

She first got mental health care at age sixteen, only after her mother, a nurse's tech, "was riding my ass about something, and I told her to get out of my face, and she kept persisting, and I pushed her," she recalled. "My dad saw me push her, and they ended up both on top of me; he held my arms down while she beat the hell out of me. So, my parents deemed at that point that I had to be crazy. Not crazy in the sense of a diagnosed disorder, but that I was too different from the family unit to coexist with them."

She was sent to an inpatient behavioral health facility for teens where she got therapy and antidepressants. She stayed for five months, much of her junior year, then came home and finished high school. Even while using pot, cocaine, and ecstasy, and binge drinking several times a week, she did well enough to get a scholarship to Austin Peay State University in nearby Clarksville.

During this time, she also married a man five years older than she was. The marriage didn't last long. She ended up dropping out of college during her freshman year and then training as a bartender.

"So, I'm an eighteen-year-old bartender," she explained, "and I'm drinking on the job all the time. One day these two guys came in while I was working. They stayed pretty late, and at the end of the night they asked if I did drugs. I said I did, and they asked, 'Have you ever free-based?' I had never heard of it. I didn't know what it was."

She went with them to their car and tried smoking crack for the first time. "It was absolutely amazing," she recalled. "It was almost like it transformed my idea of getting high, because I'd never been so high in my life. And I mean, it's just out of control, but I was able to function at the same time. I cleared out my bank account that night, over $1,000. I had to take it out $300 at a time because that's all the ATM would let me draw. And I just spent it on crack just like that."

This began a period in her life where she was largely homeless, couch-surfing: "I'm basically sleeping with people for a place to stay," she recalled. For a while she just smoked crack and occasionally heroin. And then she was introduced to intravenous heroin.

"This guy tied me and put the needle in my arm because I didn't know how to do any of that," she explained, "and gave me a little bit and, I pretty much passed out and came to and thought, 'This is the best drug. There is no other drug better than this one.' Instantly, I did not want ecstasy or cocaine or marijuana or alcohol or any of it. Just heroin."

She and the guy who introduced her to IV heroin got into an abusive relationship. To make money for drugs, she would go into local chain bookstores, steal audiobooks (because she could get more of them into her bag than printed books), and then sell them to a used bookstore. She was arrested several times and twice spent several months in jail. Her drug use did, however, lead her to get more care.

"One day I was in the bathroom, and this guy slammed the bathroom door so hard that the whole ceiling collapsed on top of me," she said. "The globe light fixture hit me in the face because I looked up, and my face was cut all over."

Her parents found out about this because her mother worked as a nurse tech at a nearby hospital. "She saw my face and begged me to leave this guy and go into treatment," she recalled. "And I did."

She was twenty-one when she went for a twenty-eight-day detox at Elam Mental Health Center in Nashville, her care covered by a grant-based program. When she came out of the program, her parents invited her to move back in with them. They wanted to support her recovery.

Ironically, before she had been in detox, she only knew the one guy who could get her heroin. In treatment, she met others who struggled with opiates, and so had more contacts for getting drugs after she was out. It wasn't long before she was using again.

"My parents found out," she recalled, "and so, understandably, they kicked me out."

For money, she started doing some sex work for an escort service. "It wasn't like an extreme case where I was being beaten or the madam was taking all my money or anything like that," she explained. "I met this woman, she was an older lady, real short, they call her 'Little Debbie' on the streets. And she had a lot of clientele and just wanted the benefit of my younger looks. I'd never done anything like that before. But it wasn't a new, surprising thing. It actually felt normal. I'd been having sex since I was twelve. And I'd always use sex to kind of get what I wanted. It felt like the next natural thing to get money for it. And I thought I was being very safe about it. You know, I would use protection, and I would validate people's driver's licenses. But the reality is all of these people were strangers."

She did this escort work on and off, through her early and mid-twenties. It gave her enough financial stability to go back to college, where she started studying psychology, business, and writing. But she would still binge on drugs and end up at the emergency room of Vanderbilt University Hospital or another Nashville hospital. According to her records, she had ten emergency admissions at Vanderbilt in 2011, another seven in 2012. Sometimes she came in after making a suicide attempt with pills; other times she would appear at the emergency department completely paranoid, with cuts on her arms, explaining that bacteria was under her skin and in her bloodstream, and the only solution was to cut herself to get it out.

She didn't have the money to pay for care beyond the emergency room, which couldn't turn her down. She worked part-time at McDonald's and had a generous friend in Nashville who would pay some of her medical bills in cash if she couldn't get assistance. She was able to feed herself largely because of the Supplemental Nutrition Assistance Program, from which she could get benefits for up to six months at a time.

"I was trying to get my life somewhat stable," she recalled, "but I was very indigent."

DURING THIS TIME, Ashley was connected to a Vanderbilt-trained psychiatrist, a woman who looked at her case from a different perspective. And after years of mostly being seen as someone who needed to be in recovery from drugs and alcohol use—somebody whose main problem was self-control and willpower—she began exploring the possibility that her underlying, or at least co-occurring, problem was a psychiatric illness. The psychiatrist began asking more detailed questions about her auditory and visual hallucinations and realized that while Ashley had them when high or intoxicated, she also had them when she was sober. So, while the hallucinations could be exacerbated by her addictive behaviors, they didn't go away even when she was in long-term recovery.

This psychiatrist was the first to suggest that Ashley suffered from schizoaffective disorder, bipolar type—an illness that combines some of the mood features of bipolar depression and some of the hallucinations and disordered thoughts of schizophrenia. The illness does often respond to medication and supportive talk therapy. Ashley was just happy to know that what she experienced wasn't entirely unusual and that it hadn't been caused by her drug use.

"This told me that I wasn't just *broken,* y'know," she said. "It gave me some hope that with medication and proper treatment it could be fixed." But the treatment wasn't easy, and some of the medication was sedating and made it hard to concentrate on her classes. She was taking lithium, as well as what was then a relatively new and expensive antipsychotic, lurasidone (Latuda), for which there was, at the time, no generic available. (When new drugs come on the market, they are only available in more expensive "brand name" form; this means some patients won't be able to easily access them unless their physicians specifically request them and the patient can handle the higher co-pay.)

In 2013, when she was twenty-six, she was transferred from the emergency department of another hospital to Vanderbilt in really bad shape. According to her charts (which she gave her physician permission to discuss with me for the book), she was admitted with "worsening paranoia, PTSD, and suicidal ideation" with a "plan to slice her veins . . . because she needed to cut out the bacteria under her skin, because not all of it bled out." She was also seeing and hearing "shadow people."

She had already cut herself, but not so badly that it required stitches. She told the doctors that she was not suicidal, and her tox screen only showed evidence of pot and benzodiazepine, so she had not used heroin or crack cocaine. She said she had been taking Latuda for a while but didn't think it was helping her symptoms anymore.

After being stabilized successfully, Ashley was able to apply for Medicare and Social Security disability, so she didn't have to keep selling drugs, or her body, for money. She ended up going to a long-term residential treatment facility, Turning Point, in southern Georgia, and when she finished, she was able to stay sober for a while through twelve-step meetings and return to college. But eventually, she started using again and dropped out of school.

For a period, she lived outdoors, in one of several tent cities set up in the Nashville area, especially Brookmeade Park in West Nashville, which is in the woods next to the Cumberland River, not far from a Walmart and a Lowe's. She was able to remain sober for periods of up to nine months, and then usually would get depressed, use crack again to buoy her spirits, end up in the hospital and detox, and then start again. People in twelve-step focus strongly on how long they have been sober, beginning the clock over every time they relapse. Ashley kept track of how long she had not taken individual drugs—heroin, crack—as well as how long she was free from all drug use.

She worked in grocery stores, she got work cleaning houses, and she did other odd jobs. When she could, she attended writing workshops.

When she was feeling well, she also volunteered to help feed unhoused people in the tent cities where she had once lived and brought them antibiotics and other medicines. She made sure they had plenty of the small nasal spray bottles of naloxone (Narcan), the drug used to revive people during opioid overdoses by blocking their opiate receptors.

In 2019, after three years away from opiates, one of her friends in the Brookemeade Park tent city offered her heroin during a visit. For some reason, she said yes. She overdosed in a way she never had before.

Her friend ran and got the naloxone that Ashley had brought and sprayed a dose into Ashley's nose. Two long minutes passed, and Ashley didn't wake up. So she was given a second dose up her nose. Then a third. But she was still unconscious.

Giving a person more naloxone than they need won't harm them. The fourth dose finally revived her. As soon as she was conscious, she went to Vanderbilt Hospital and checked herself in for psychiatric treatment, as she had so many times before.

THIS TIME, THE HOSPITAL had just recently received federal funding, as a response to the opioid crisis—especially important because Tennessee was one of the states that turned down federal Medicaid expansion—for an ambitious new approach to patients who chronically relapsed, based on ideas from the relatively new medical subspecialty of "addiction psychiatry." Dr. David Marcovitz, Vanderbilt's young director of addiction psychiatry, led the effort to use the funding to rethink their approach to care for patients exactly like Ashley, to basically use staff physicians, teaching clinics, nurse practitioners, social workers, and recovery coaches to offer completely integrated care and what are called "wrap-around supports." The idea was that most of the cracks that patients fell through—between inpatient hospitalization, intensive outpatient care, and normal outpatient care; between addiction and psychiatric care; between medical and nonmedical care; between peer support for recovery and ongoing psychiatric care—would be, if not perfectly filled, then at least aggressively addressed, as proactively as possible, by an addiction consult service and a transitional outpatient bridge clinic.

Ashley was the ideal patient for this approach. She was considered a unique case, both in terms of the sheer number of her serious mental health and substance use emergencies and her ability to function in the daily world, go to college, and have what appeared to be genuine insight into her condition. She also had astonishing resilience. No matter how ill she was when she came in, she was always somehow "the right amount of agreeable," in the words of one of her doctors there. And she always left with an optimistic attitude, a path ahead, hope.

But she had a tendency to disappear from regular outpatient psychotherapy. She would stop taking her meds or, worse, take them too quickly, especially the meds she was given to counteract sedation.

And she had almost no experience with the growing world of MAT (medication-assisted treatment) for addiction. There were several newer, powerful medications that could be used to help control a patient's desire for drugs or alcohol in one of two ways. Naltrexone (Vivitrol) blocked the effects of drugs and alcohol so they no longer caused "highs." Buprenorphine (Suboxone) reduced cravings by replacing some of the effects of drugs or alcohol, but at a much lower level. They were controversial in traditional recovery circles, just as the original long-term treatment for heroin use, methadone (Methadose), always had been—because they were seen as forms of substitute addiction, while abstinence supported by twelve-step meetings was considered the only real long-term solution.

Like most people with substance use disorders—myself included—Ashley had only ever been prescribed buprenorphine or naltrexone in the hospital during the first week, or weeks, of detox. They were never offered to her as long-term maintenance options, and her one experience on methadone had been miserable: "I didn't like to stand in line at six o'clock in the morning every day," she explained. "It felt like going to a drug dealer."

But now MAT use was being expanded, and more physicians were able to write prescriptions for the medications. Vanderbilt was part of that cutting-edge treatment. Yet even with these innovations in addiction psychiatry, Ashley had what her doctor called "complex, coexisting disorders" that required judgment calls balancing psychiatric meds and MAT.

"In most places," her doctor said, "if you want to get Suboxone and psychiatric care at the same clinic, good luck!" But even with that integrated approach, a case like Ashley's is complicated. "You want to put your nickel down on an underlying disorder versus substance-induced symptoms, and it's challenging. Also, it's rare that a patient would stick with it, and be so open to trying all these different parts of our continuum of care. It's not unheard of, but she's one of only a handful of patients who have been able to stick with it—despite the kind of stumbling she still experiences."

As HER HEALTH slowly improved, Ashley started her own business acting as a health-care aide to some elderly Nashville residents. One of her therapists at Vanderbilt also convinced her that she needed to start finding more people who had similar interests. At a local library, she noticed there was a writer's group being held there. She was interested in learning more about creative nonfiction, so she went to the class. The facilitator of the group was Drew Dunlop, a big, intensely kind guy with a shaved head, twenty-two years older than she was, with an MBA and a partly finished MFA, but also his own health challenges. He had schizoaffective disorder and a history of suicidal depression, although his symptoms were under much better control than hers. He liked her and her writing, and they went out on a couple of dates. Then COVID hit, Drew thought he might have it, and they decided to quarantine together.

"When you quarantine with someone, you find out real quick whether you get along with them or not," Ashley said. They fell in love; his nickname for her was "Sweets." Drew had experience getting psychiatric help—both inpatient and outpatient—but also giving psychological help: he had worked as an adolescent substance abuse counselor in a variety of settings and was working toward his master's in mental health counseling. But none of that entirely prepared him for having a girlfriend who, periodically, would just disappear for several hours, or sometimes for several days, using meth, and when her meth dealer got busted, using crack, and then either coming home or calling from the emergency room.

The first couple of times it happened, he went out looking for her, to try to rescue her. But, to Ashley, that was even worse. She was upset and angry that Drew would put himself in danger for her—more danger than she felt like she was in, because she knew how to handle herself in these situations. She finally convinced Drew that when she left, he needed to just wait at home for her. He would text her; sometimes she would text back. And, while waiting, he would think about all the advice he had given people in addiction counseling—both the patients and their families—and search for a version of it that worked for him and Ashley.

He also wondered sometimes if maybe "everything I told them was crap."

Drew developed a unique way of seeing their situation. "I trust Ashley one hundred percent," he told me. "And I trust the addiction not at all. I never refer to it as 'her addiction.' It's 'the addiction" and I don't see her in the addiction. When she's relapsing, I only think of it in terms of the addiction. I don't take it personally at all. It's not like she's doing this to hurt me. I know that a woman without money has no problem getting drugs. That's just reality. I have this duality in my head that if she slept with somebody to get drugs, she could confide that to me and I wouldn't be hurt by that. But if she slept with somebody because of fun, or because she wanted a better emotional or sexual connection, then I'd be devastated. But it all goes back to this: I separate Ashley from the addiction.

"Once, she disappeared, with just an occasional text, for about sixty hours. And I only got half an hour's sleep during that time, trying to control her, to get her to come back, through text messages, saying, 'You can do it, I know,' and everything. While I'm waiting for her, I'm binge-watching *Breaking Bad* but somehow it never even connected with me that I was *living it.* So, I was really in despair.

"I am very concerned when she relapses because she has died and been revived. Because the thing is, if she dies, hospitals won't tell you if she's there. And nobody that is with her has any idea how to contact me, if they would even bother to contact me. So, she could all of a sudden, you know, she could overdose and die. And then I may not know for days or even a week or whatever."

Their first year together navigating this was the first year of COVID. They got engaged in June 2020 and married in late February 2021. "Probably the most heartbreaking thing we've been through," Drew said, "was the day of our wedding. It was a beautiful day. And then in the evening she said, 'I really need to go get drugs. I've been fighting it for two or three weeks.' And I asked her not to. But she said, 'I'll be right back' and she went and got meth on our wedding night and ingested it."

Drew paused, looked away, and pursed his lips: "Now, you're the first person I've told that." It wasn't, he said, because he was embarrassed by it. He just "didn't want anyone to judge Ashley."

WHILE ASHLEY AND DREW were pleased with the unique wraparound care program at Vanderbilt, neither they nor their doctors were satisfied with how well they helped her prevent relapses. For the past couple of years, she has been taking lithium, the antipsychotic medication aripiprazole (Abilify)—initially in the form of a monthly shot, until it started wearing off too early and she switched to the pill form—as well as a low dose of the anti-addiction medication Suboxone.

She was also given the stimulant lisdexamfetamine (Vyvanse) to help her concentration and to control sedation; while technically not a stimulant, it is still a controlled substance, and not every practice would give it to a patient with a history of addiction. But Ashley has a history of good insight into her illness and not abusing her prescription meds, so they considered it a risk worth taking—with extra oversight. Drew held her stimulant for her, just in case. (For my personal care, I go to a psychiatrist with training from the American Society of Addiction Medicine just to make sure he can make these kinds of judgment calls.)

When going back over relapses in her mind, Ashley said she believed the beginning of each process was some breakthrough depression. To kick-start her flagging mood, she began to "jump my Vyvanse"—meaning she asked Drew for more each day than she was supposed to take and ran out of it more quickly. Then she might start seeking small amounts of cocaine, so when she went to Vanderbilt for her regular drug screen, she let them know she was likely to test positive. But they couldn't give her more Vyvanse if she tested positive.

So this cycle sometimes led her to binge on meth or crack for a couple of days.

In the fall of 2022, she found herself in one of these cycles. Then, one of her health-care aide clients, who she had known for eight years and cared for weekly over the past two, died suddenly. Christmas was approaching and, as is true for many, the holidays were hard for Ashley. It was her late mother's favorite holiday, so "I now dread Christmas, it's not a time for family for me anymore, it's empty. Spiritually it has the same meaning, but as far as fellowship and family, it's not the same at all." Her seventy-two-year-old father was the only one left in the family she remained in contact with. And for much of the past twenty years, he had never really supported or understood her treatment.

To try to get ahead of these kindling symptoms, she was shifted from weekly outpatient talk therapy to IOP—the intensive outpatient program—which met three times a week at night and offered more support. But then she got in trouble trying to help a homeless man who attended the group and carried a gun in his backpack for protection on the streets. She told him to put his backpack in the trunk of her car during the session. Police came looking for him for some reason after a session, which eventually led them to her car. She didn't get in trouble, but she was excused from the IOP.

"I threw up my hands, and said, 'I'll show you, I'll hurt myself right now,'" she told me. Ashley went directly to a nearby park, bought cocaine, and began smoking it. For the next several days, she bought and used hundreds of dollars' worth of cocaine. She was also sexually assaulted. One of her regular dealers was a gang member who had never given her any trouble before. But this time he had in tow a young man who wanted to join the gang. He was instructed to rape Ashley.

"It was his initiation," she recalled. "They targeted me because they saw me, every day, come through there to get cocaine. I'm just grateful that I didn't die, 'cause they could have easily killed me and thrown me in the dumpster." She didn't report the attack because she feared retaliation when she returned to the park. It was one of her regular places to buy drugs.

She finally ended up at the emergency department of Vanderbilt University Hospital and was admitted for a seven-day detox.

One night her father came to visit her at the hospital. He had seemed a little different toward her recently. He would occasionally ask Drew a question or two about her health, and he seemed to have maybe done a little research on the internet. That night the three of them were sitting together in the family room in the addiction care unit, a place where bad news was often shared. The nurses had just finished their meeting in the room, and then Ashley and Drew and her dad came in and found chairs.

After sitting quietly for a bit, Ashley's dad turned to her and, out of the blue, said the most surprising thing.

"I'm startin' to think," he said, "that this thing . . . is a *disease* that you have."

She and Drew were both stunned. "It was the first time I realized that he sees this as a real thing," she said. "It's not something that I'm faking, not something I'm doing for *attention*. This is a real issue that I live with *every day*."

What did you say to him?

"I can't recall," she said. "I think I was too amazed to say anything."

SHE GOT OUT of detox, stayed sober for a few weeks, and then started using again. She and Drew were feeling desperate. They decided she needed another inpatient stay, the second in five weeks, but it was time to try something different.

They also decided it was time to try some*where* different—hoping that a change of scenery, away from a city she knew so well, might be helpful. One of her drug dealers had begun very aggressively harassing and threatening Drew and her—on the phone, by text, even showing up at the house.

But, in a larger sense, the whole city of Nashville now seemed like a trigger to her, a place where it was too easy to relapse. "I've been staring at that skyline for twenty years," she said, "especially because a lot of times when I smoke crack, it's in a place called 'fifteenth tower'—because it's on the fifteenth floor of a housing project called Park Tower. We go up there and when we're smoking, we see the whole skyline of Nashville. So, I associate the skyline with using. Period. Every time I come into the city, whether it be on 65 South from Kentucky, I get right over the edge and there's the skyline. And the first thing I think is, 'Man, I'd love a hit right now.' I have too much emotional connection to that city."

So, they decided she would do her twenty-eight-day inpatient treatment at Rivendell Behavioral Health Hospital in Bowling Green, Kentucky, about sixty-five miles away from home. And she insisted on doing it without the help of detox medications, so full-on withdrawal. At Rivendell, it was recommended that Ashley go into a long inpatient stay—six months or longer—which she had done when she was younger but never with the new approaches to addiction psychiatry and recovery.

There was only one problem—there was no place in Tennessee or Kentucky that would take Medicaid and treat her anytime soon. She was told she might have to wait a year.

Also, because she was now in Kentucky, the doctors and staff who had been supporting her and Drew at Vanderbilt could no longer, technically, help them. The funding for their innovative program didn't allow their care to cross the state line. (The director of the program told me they would have tried to help them, at least in decision-making, but Ashley and Drew assumed they could not and didn't reach out.)

The only place she could find that would take her insurance and consider her for long-term care was two states away in Louisiana. Even though she and Drew were good at researching options (and Ashley has been at a number of local places before), they only had access to so much up-to-date information through Google searches and internet reviews.

This is a huge part of the problem with care—when someone finally reaches the point where they will commit to a major, possibly life-changing program, there is often no simple way to find one with an opening that will accept your insurance. Every state has its own rules and coverage, only for people who live in that state. Each care facility is entrepreneurial in its own way, and many are unaffiliated with larger medical systems. You pretty much need a concierge medical consultant for you and your family to make the best decision at that crucial moment, one who knows the strengths and weaknesses of different programs and facilities, as well as the details of your illness and finances. While there are individual people with this kind of knowledge for different regions—sometimes accessed through hospital social work staff, sometimes from knowledgeable people in support groups—what is needed is better consumer information that helps people and their families navigate state lines and laws.

So, Ashley decided to do a long stay in a "sober living house," which she had never tried before because most of them were so closely tied to the hard-core AA/twelve-step world, less integrated with psychiatry than her care had been. She had been in all kinds of rehab centers for the standard twenty-eight days but had never shared a house with other people supporting each other's sobriety, actively working the twelve steps, and being regularly drug tested. They decided to try this in Kentucky.

Ashley and Drew became a long-distance couple. She would come home for a day on the weekends from the sober living house in Kentucky, where she lived with fourteen other recovering women. The house was very old-school twelve-step, and Ashley didn't really talk about the addiction medication she takes because she knew some would hassle her about that. Her sponsor there knew she was being treated medically as well, but her main focus, on a daily basis, was working the steps and working to stay sober so she could return to living with Drew.

She was also thinking more about how she might need to rely on twelve-step meetings for daily support if she started going off her meds to try to get pregnant. This is a common challenge for all women of childbearing age—balancing how safe it is for a baby if the mother is taking psychiatric medicine versus how safe it is for the mother to go off her medication. None of the drugs Ashley takes are actually prohibited for pregnant mothers. But there are risks of taking them, especially the Suboxone, which specifically addresses her cravings for opiates. Some babies have been born with distress, leading them to be temporarily treated for withdrawal.

"I want to have a family," she said, "but I will not put a newborn through withdrawal."

THE NEXT TIME I talked to Ashley, she was home on a day pass from the sober living house, sitting in her living room with Drew, wearing his oversize red NPR T-shirt and excited about how long she had been sober. She wanted me to know she had gotten her AA ninety-day chip. She and Drew were so proud.

Not long after, I heard from Drew that Ashley had relapsed on her ninety-fifth day. Drew described the episode partly clinically and partly emotionally. "She was active for four or so days," he wrote, "and was letting her world burn down." Normally, a relapse would have forced her to leave the sober living house, but Ashley was such a unique case, with unique social and medical support, and she was so well-liked in the house, that they made a rare exception and allowed her to return after a week of hospitalization. She also was able to keep her job after disappearing for a week because her boss came to understand it was due to a medical condition.

Ashley and Drew both felt very positive that this recent setback was a turning point. Drew noted that when he picked her up to take her to the hospital, she still had a small amount of crack but, for the first time ever, she didn't finish it.

"She threw about twenty dollars' worth of the crack, and her crack pipe and push stick, out the window," he told me. "That was a huge demonstration of how serious she was."

At the same time, while Drew was excited about having a baby with Ashley, he was always realistic about what could happen. "Ashley has said she would never use while pregnant, and definitely not use while she had a child to take care of," he explained. "However, I've told her that addiction doesn't ask your permission to fuck up your life, so we can't take that for granted. And this knowledge gave me reason to give deep consideration to whether we have children. I first asked myself if I wanted to have kids at my age, and it only took a short time to say yes. Then I asked myself if I wanted them with her, and that took zero seconds to say yes. But then came the really important question: 'Am I willing and prepared to raise a child alone if Ashley should relapse and disappear and/or die?' This took a few days of consideration, but I finally said yes and now have no reservation about this. I think it is important for people in my position to ask themselves these questions when considering having children with people whose addiction is in remission. It is sad, but having to raise a child or children alone is a very real possibility, and if they're not ready to do it, they should give that heavy consideration. We must avoid a delusional belief that the addict/alcoholic would 'never do that' when it comes to relapsing while being a parent."

They decided their best strategy would be if they gave up their place in Nashville, and Drew would move to Bowling Green—so she could remain in sober living there, keep her job, and the couple could be together. They found a great house not far from the serene Barren River, put a nonrefundable deposit down on it, and gave notice to their current landlord. They were just about to move when Ashley relapsed again, this time for five straight days, after which it was recommended that she do a long-term inpatient rehab for the first time in years. There wasn't a bed available for her in Kentucky or Tennessee; the only place that would take her was Turning Point in Georgia, where she had been ten years earlier.

This was the first time she had ever gone away to rehab by plane, by herself, and when Drew was saying goodbye to her at the airport, while they were laughing and smiling, he found himself thinking, "Am I seeing her for the last time?" She flew to Tallahassee, where she and another new patient, a very drunk fellow, were picked up and driven one hundred miles to the facility. She planned to stay there for six months.

Drew was stunned to find himself not only suddenly alone but forced to move days later to Bowling Green. Friends helped him move and many of them donated to a GoFundMe page they created to help cover the expense. He was trying to figure out when he might be able to visit Ashley once she finished detox and had settled in for her long stay. But, within weeks, the couple reached out to let me know that Ashley had left Turning Point.

"All too often," Ashley told me, "rehabilitation centers will offer many things on their website but will deliver a completely ridiculous regimen for therapy. There were many groups at Turning Point that consisted of coloring, and watching TED Talks or Disney movies. I was not satisfied with the quality of my care."

After discussing this with several twelve-step friends in Kentucky, including her sponsor, Ashley had called Drew and asked him to come pick her up. He made the nine-hour drive down to Turning Point, Ashley got in the car, and they turned around and drove straight back. Ashley got to spend her first night in the house in Bowling Green that she and Drew had rented, and he had been living in alone.

Ashley had reached out to her doctors at Vanderbilt who told her to remain in touch and they would be available if she wanted to return to their care. For insurance reasons, however, she chose a new therapist in Kentucky instead and felt she was making breakthroughs on processing some of her early childhood traumas.

She was going to AA meetings every day and had a new sponsor she talked to every day. "I'm a ball of anxiety," she said, "but meditation for about ten minutes several times throughout the day helps me exercise focus." She was also writing and drawing every day and taking photographs.

She sent me a couple of beautiful shots of the lush, peaceful river she got to look at every day.

"Seems to be going smoothly right now," she said.

NOBODY I'VE MET during this book has been through as many changes, and endured so many catastrophic relapses, as Ashley Dunlop. I'm amazed by her ability to survive her own illness and the stunning resilience of her marriage. And each time she returns, I'm reminded of a letter Drew shared with me, which he wrote to her hoping both to inspire her and maybe to scare her a little—because he knows that after every relapse, the first question she asks is, "Are you still with me?"

My Sweets,

Love flows from my heart for you at twilight and dusk, and all the moments in between. It is yours in your presence and your absence, when you're lucid and when you're high, in both your sickness and in your health. It is undying, unending, unwavering . . .

I can bear much more for you, for my love, commitment, and duty demand it. But my dearest lady, I don't want to bear it anymore. I am tired. I am tired of fear for your health, for your safety, for your life. I am tired of fear for our future, for our children, for the life we have always imagined we wanted and which we both richly deserve . . .

I have never demanded anything of you in strong terms, but it is best for you, me, and us that I do so now; I demand you choose our life and say a permanent goodbye to the one that keeps seducing you, the one leading you to the death of your dignity, of your life, of your beautiful soul. I demand you cast aside the distorted beliefs that you deserve degradation, destruction, death.

And I demand from now on that you only wake up after falling asleep, not come to after passing out.

I will take those strong demands and now convert them to gentle requests. Sweets, please do these things for you. Do them for me. Do them for us.

With eternal, limitless love,

Your True

Chapter Seven

Cousin Harry

When we decided that a book of profiles of people living with mental illnesses should include at least one who had lost the struggle, I immediately thought of my twenty-two-year-old Texas cousin Harry McMurrey. A handsome, exuberant cowboy and golfer—who saw the world as a dance floor he was always ready to leap onto—Harry died by suicide in 2017, in the spring of his senior year in college.

I will never forget the memorial service for him. It was held at St. Barnabas Episcopal Church in tiny Fredericksburg, Texas, not far from the family ranch where Harry and his younger siblings lived. Harry was the son of my cousin Mark McMurrey—whose mother is my mom's sister—and his ex-wife Ceci.

The place was jammed, not only with family from across the country but also Harry's college classmates. He had attended the University of the South in Sewanee, Tennessee, where he had been a captain of the highly ranked golf team, and a boy-most-likely, with so much ahead of him. And then, the summer before his senior year, he suffered a concussion at the family ranch when a calf ran him into a metal fencepost. The incident seemingly triggered a series of changes and declines until early February, when he called his father from college and told him he needed to withdraw immediately. "I can't stay here one more day," Harry had said, although he didn't really explain why.

I remember Mark standing up to get ready to approach the podium and eulogize his firstborn child. I also rose to hug him as hard as I could, whispering into his ear, "There was nothing wrong with Harry. He died of a disease. It manifests itself in a terrible way, but it's still a disease."

It was, frankly, the first and last time we talked about what happened to Harry until recently. The fact that he had taken his own life wasn't mentioned during the funeral, or in the obituary, or by anybody in the family. Mark's ex-wife and kids are more religious than he is, and I heard a lot of people say Harry's death was "God's will." But I never heard that from Mark.

Yet, when I asked Mark to speak to me about Harry for this book, it was as if seven years of pent-up emotion came flooding out. What was fascinating to me, and to Mark, was just how little they knew about what had happened to Harry, and how little what they knew had been processed in any helpful way. It was all still so raw.

I've had more powerful conversations with my cousin Mark about all of this than we've ever shared in our lives. I was also able to speak at great length with Harry's younger brother Belton, a filmmaker, and with one of Harry's best friends from college. Harry's sister Estella, a college student, did speak with me, but then asked me not to use our conversation (an option I gave to anyone interviewed for this book). Harry's mother, Ceci, chose not to speak to me about this.

The value of exploring the aftermath of a suicide is not to bring the person back but to learn lessons that may help those who are still here and struggling, as well as their families. I think it's important to do even if that exploration is hard for people who have experienced the losses. I also believe it is never too late to ask out loud the big questions that have been welling up inside since you first got that call.

For Mark, that came at nine-thirty in the morning as he was standing behind his desk in his Austin office. And when he heard the news from his ex-wife, he told me, "I just fell on the ground." He was so distracted he rushed out without saying anything to his friend in the next office, who had lost a child just two years earlier himself. Mark hurried home, picked up what he would need for the funeral, and started driving west toward Fredericksburg. He called another friend who also had lost his own daughter to suicide the year before.

Mark recalled his friend saying, "First of all, I don't know if you should be driving, but if you feel like you're okay, we just have to get you there." Then, as they started talking, he stopped Mark and said, "It's way too early for you to hear this, but I'll say it anyway. The very second you quit trying to explain *why* this happened is the moment you're going to start getting better."

Yet all Mark could think about was: Why? Had he and Ceci lost their son, and Belton and Estella their brother, because of head trauma, because of mental illness, or because of something else? Had anybody—including Harry—understood what was wrong with him or how ill he was? Harry was pretty religious; he had received both medical and faith-based pastoral care after his concussion. What role had religion and spirituality played?

When I tried to comfort Mark by saying it was "a disease," did I really know what disease? Is being suicidal a symptom of a disease? Is it a disease itself? And are these questions different for families and public health officials trying to prevent suicide and for those trying to make sense of losses to suicide?

As he kept driving, Mark called the Austin psychiatrist he had taken Harry to see the day he came home from school and who had been treating him for depression since.

"He was crushed to hear this," Mark told me. "He also said Harry was 'not somebody I thought was going to harm himself. He was not on my radar as someone who would hurt himself.' So, for me to hear that when, well, the reason he came home in the first place was because he said he was going to harm himself. For the doctor to say he wasn't on the radar . . ."

Mark paused for a second: "My comment to him, and I don't mean to be flip about this, was, 'If he wasn't on your radar, then we need a bigger radar screen.'"

MY COUSIN MARK is an Austin business development consultant who grew up, as I did, in a family with a mom who had an alcohol use disorder, and later became extremely engaged with AA. Mark remembered his mother—my mom's younger sister, Candy—first checking into a facility in Houston when he was a junior in college at UT Austin. His father was in recovery as well. Their friends in Texas never really understood. "I later became friends with some of my parents' friends," he explained, "and they would always say, 'Your parents used to be so much fun. They were big partiers and everybody loved them. Does that really mean they were, you know, alcoholic?' And the answer is yes: I've found my dad passed out in the driveway in his car."

My mother had similar experiences. Their family, the Bennetts, had a powerful genetic predisposition to alcohol use. Their mother, maternal grandmother to Mark and me, was the most ill. Mark remembered his family going on a very depressing visit to her Cocoa

Beach apartment when he was around thirteen. Just a few weeks later, she was found dead in her shower, having been there for days. She was only sixty-five.

Mark and his siblings were always close with my brother, sister, and me. His family would come to the Cape in the summer; he was interested in golf, having grown up in Texas, while we were more interested in sailing, having grown up in Boston and Hyannis. But, as he said, "I assimilated pretty easily, especially since I was a golfer and the dads all wanted to play golf."

After college, Mark went into real estate finance in Houston, and then his company moved him to California because the market was better. While he did some drugs and drinking in college—tempered by the fact that he was an athlete and had to be able to perform in golf and other sports—by his midtwenties he found himself in L.A. with a number of our family members, some of whom were already in recovery. In fact, my mom and his mom had helped many of them get into recovery.

"Since all the members of my immediate family were in AA," Mark told me, "I decided I should try it." So he committed to the standard ninety meetings in ninety days (which is how everyone is supposed to start twelve-step treatment). "Sometimes we went to, well, let's just call it the Hollywood meeting," he said, "which is like going to a cocktail party without the cocktails, and there are dozens of people there, many of whom you would know." He also accompanied one of his friends to a hospital to help a fellow AA member "and you see this guy is literally handcuffed to a bed, and he's gonna go to jail after he gets detoxed from whatever he was on, but my friend was preaching to him—so that actually counted as a meeting. I literally went to every kind of meeting you can think of."

While he didn't stay in AA, he understood the attraction of a sober life. "I had friends I'd be playing pickup basketball with down in Venice Beach," he recalled, "hanging out and these were seriously sober guys. They had a very strict lifestyle."

So, Mark grew up in a world that did not pay a lot of attention to psychiatry but rather viewed people's problems more through the prism of substance use disorders and the need for abstinence. It was hard-core AA, extremely behavioral: you drank because you were an alcoholic, and you stopped drinking by going to meetings, working the steps, humbling yourself to the higher power. "Mental health" was something else altogether.

In 1991, Mark married Cecilia Johnson, whose father, B.K., was heir to the largest ranch in Texas, King Ranch in south Texas near Corpus Christi—but also created his own ranch and empire closer to San Antonio. B.K. was a legendary hunter and drinker; the euphemism used by the family when he got drunk was that "he would get spun up."

"Since my ex-wife is from one of the wealthier families in Texas, I then had a source of investable funds," Mark explained. He left the company he was working for and "we agreed to live our life trying to build businesses around stuff that we were interested in together." They initially lived together in California, but when Ceci was pregnant, they moved back to Texas, and Harry was born in Austin in 1995. His middle name was the family name of my aunt and my mother: Bennett.

When Harry was nine months old, they took a trip to New Zealand for the winter holidays. On January 2 they got news that a family member was being checked into addiction treatment in Minnesota, and they flew back to be there for the first family meeting. It was the beginning of another generation of both families growing up in AA and recovery culture. "With all four grandparents having alcohol issues," he noted, "the kids knew all about treatment because even when people weren't in the throes of it, they heard about it." Mark and Ceci moved to San Antonio, where they had another son, Belton, in 1997, and a daughter, Estella, in 2000.

Ceci's father died in 2001, when Harry was six. While he left his children and grandchildren some money, the bulk of his estate was left to his third wife. This led to a massive court case in which Mark and Ceci were actively involved; they and other family members claimed there had been major changes in B.K.'s will after he had lost mental capacity to alcoholism. The case would drag on for over a decade. It became, in a way, one of those businesses Mark and Ceci were in together.

In 2004, the couple bought a piece of property outside of Fredericksburg, population 11,000—about seventy miles west of Austin—which they hoped to develop into a ranch home and winery. While building a guesthouse on the property, they stayed thirty miles away at another family ranch, Chinquapin, in Mountain Home. A year later, the family moved to the new ranch, dubbed "Divina," and the kids began attending Fredericksburg schools. Harry was in middle school when they moved.

IT WASN'T LONG before Mark and Ceci separated. It was a relatively amicable split but was still, as Belton told me, a challenge for him and his siblings, the impact of which he and Harry talked about more as they got older. In 2007, when Harry was twelve, Mark moved to a house "in town" in Fredericksburg so he could see the kids as often as possible. Harry and his siblings lived on the ranch with their mother and split weekends between their parents' places.

Belton said that growing up, he viewed Harry as being closer to, and more like, their father: "handsome, charming, charismatic guys . . . and both had aggressive and, very frankly, impatient personalities." Belton was closer to and more like their mother, "an English major" who was more "bookish" and "spiritual," and committed to raising her kids on a ranch. (In 2015, when Harry was in college, Mark moved to Austin—more than an hour away—and the kids stayed with him there on weekends.)

Harry grew up to be a charming, engaging young man who, under Mark's guidance, developed an excellent golf game. He practiced golf, he played golf, he exercised for golf, he watched golf tournaments and documentaries, he thought golf. He put a lot into golf and expected a lot from it.

Besides golf, Harry loved ranching and dressed the part: whenever he could, he wore a cowboy hat. He worked several summers at the family ranch and developed into a good cowboy—enduring long days of tough, physical work, which he enjoyed. He was an excellent rider, knew how to rope, and was a great shot. And he worked diligently, often up at 5:00 A.M. to do work on the far side of the ranch. He was also a volunteer fireman.

Wherever he was, he loved music and dancing. When he first got his driver's license, all he wanted to do was drive around and listen to music.

As his younger sister would say in an online interview for a mental health app, "Every girl wanted to marry him, every guy wanted to be best friends with him, everybody wanted to be Harry."

Harry left for college in 2013. Instead of going somewhere in-state—pretty common for Texans—he chose the University of the South, which is usually just referred to by its location, "Sewanee," in south-central Tennessee. A private Episcopal liberal arts college established just a few years before the Civil War, every aspect of life there is rich in tradition and contradictions. Sewanee is, for example, known for its school of theology while also having a reputation for being a Christian party school.

It is also a golfer's paradise, with an utterly stunning golf course that is regularly ranked among the top fifteen college courses in the nation, and, given the climate, is playable nearly every day.

Garrett Laurie met Harry on the first day of their freshman year. Garrett was from Montgomery, Alabama, where it felt like he knew everybody, and when he arrived at Sewanee it felt like he didn't know anybody. He met Harry in the dorm hallway, and from that first time he heard Harry say "What's up, dude" in his South Texas drawl with an easy smile, Garrett knew they would be friends. They both played golf and hunted but, most important, Harry was magnetic. He hadn't been at school any longer than Garrett, but he already seemed to be friends with everyone.

"He couldn't go anywhere without saying hello," Garrett told me. "The 'passing hello' is a tradition at Sewanee, but he made it like sport. He just had no fear of meeting people. I remember the first parents weekend, my family immediately loved Harry. I'm pretty sure my dad wanted to adopt him."

Interestingly, Mark would remember that first parents weekend, which took place midfall, a little differently. It was the first time he ever saw Harry experience any kind of psychiatric symptom. In the middle of the weekend, as the family was preparing to go to a party together, Harry had a panic attack.

"I remember Ceci and I had to take turns monitoring him, and then being with the other two kids," he recalled. "They were slightly freaking out: 'Where's our brother?' And we were in kind of a big, remote area, and we couldn't have him just wandering off. We had to keep an eye on him."

They ultimately decided the panic attack "was drug-induced,"

Mark explained. "Sewanee is pretty well known for its partying. I heard they would put Xanax in the punch." But the panic attack was unusual, and out of character for Harry.

And there was also the additional pressure of joining a highly regarded college golf team.

"Harry was a great golfer," Mark said. "But there can be some issues there, because of the nature of golf being hypercompetitive. You can get down on yourself. Part of the challenge is to pick yourself back up and forget about what just happened. But it's a tough game that way."

All through junior high and high school, Mark had been Harry's golf buddy and cheerleader, and he had excelled: Harry was the captain of his school golf team, which won the Division 3A state championship during his junior year. Now he was on his own, a freshman on a major college team.

"Bad things are gonna happen on a golf course. Sometimes you might get a bad break. But that's just part of it," Mark explained. "You gotta learn that's part of the game. The way I coached him in golf—I didn't want to coach him with his swing. Because there are plenty of people that can do that, great, wonderful teachers. So, I would focus on, Okay, how do we actually play this game? How do we manage ourselves around the golf course? How do we overcome the challenge of how to compete? But it's really more about the game. And, obviously, the benefit is there are some life lessons in there, right? This sort of thing was actually really fun for us."

Harry did well on the golf team right away; in two of the four fall tournaments, he led the team or came in second by one stroke. At the second tournament of the spring season, he had a team-best 222 for three rounds; the student paper headline read "McMurrey Leads Sewanee at Jekyll Island Collegiate." He was well-liked, funny, and an endlessly engaging storyteller. And he took players under his wing to help them, on both the men's and women's teams.

Harry got the hang of college life, college parties, even college punch, and he thrived at Sewanee. Fraternity rush was second semester, and he and Garrett both got their top choice, Sigma Alpha Epsilon.

He also became more religious at college. "He would overtly say to people, 'What is your relationship with the Lord?'" Mark recalled. "This is not something most college kids say or talk about."

But it was certainly part of the ethos at Sewanee (which was also where Harry's pastor at home had gone to college). And, as Mark noted, "His mom was kind of doing the same thing. Those were her religious beliefs."

Mark respected these beliefs. But he was on a different spiritual path.

Harry's friend Garrett saw him as a "pretty spiritual guy. He always wore the Saint Christopher cross around his neck. And he had a Bible verse that he read every morning before he stepped out. After he died, his mom framed a copy of it and gave it to me for graduation. It's from Ephesians."

> I ask him to strengthen you by his spirit—not a brute strength but a glorious inner strength—that CHRIST will live in you as you open the door and invite him in. And I ask him that with both feet planted firmly on love, you'll be able to take on with all Christians the extravagant dimensions of Christ's love. Reach out and experience the breath! Test its length! Plumb the depths! Rise to the heights! Live full lives, full in the fullness of God.

In the summers, Harry loved working on the ranch. He had grown up with a King Ranch family tradition called "cousin camp." Mark explained to me, "Every year the whole family goes to the ranch and they spend a whole week together. On one of the days, the kids go in and they work the cattle. It seems quite crazily dangerous and probably is, but this is what they do and Harry loved it. It's really fun and an important part of their adult experience."

Besides the "cousin camp" week, Harry had also worked as an actual cowboy for several summers at the ranch. "Everyone saw him as someone who was really skilled," Mark said. So, there was considerable surprise when Harry got hurt at cousin camp, in June 2016, just before his senior year in college. His brother, Belton, was just a few feet away when it happened.

"Harry was 'mugging' a calf, which means he had its head in his arms and he was trying to throw it on its side," Belton recalled, "and it was just a very big calf and it threw him straight into one of the metal posts that hold up the pen. He hit his forehead and, right away, had an almost cartoonish lump on his head. I don't remember anyone ever having a head injury like that at the ranch before."

Harry was dazed but did not, as Belton recalled, ever lose consciousness. He was taken to a nearby hospital, watched overnight for additional symptoms, and diagnosed with a concussion. Mark was told that Harry was "initially dizzy and nauseous, was told to stay inside, in a dark room, not to watch TV—all the normal stuff you do with concussions. That wasn't fun during cousin camp and he missed part of that very active family week. But then it was over and we didn't think another thing about it."

While explaining this to me, Mark got quiet for a second.

"Obviously, looking back on things differently, we would have had more of a scan on his brain," he said. "Clearly, we didn't spend enough time focused on that particular thing."

But, even if nothing overt had shown up on a brain scan, there still could have been reason for increased vigilance. Studies, unfortunately not very well known at that time, already had been showing a clearer link between head injuries and the onset of mental illness. The risk was highest during the first year after a head trauma.

THAT SUMMER, BELTON recalled, Harry started to change. Until the head injury, the two brothers had been getting along better than usual—Harry was headed into his senior year in college, Belton about to leave for his freshman year at USC film school, and they had started having some more grown-up discussions about everything from the impact of their parents' divorce on their own romantic relationships to their futures. "We were really reaching a turning point in our relationship there," he recalled. "We'd be able to just go hang out after working cattle and have a beer and just chat about girls, questions about life, you know, what lies ahead."

But, after Harry's injury, Belton was away for a few weeks. And when he returned home in July, his older brother seemed different.

"It makes me uncomfortable to recall this, because I know that it probably had to do with his head trauma," Belton told me, "but he was becoming very unpleasant to be around. He was extremely impatient. Very, very aggressive in conversation. Condescending, and a little bit delusional."

He was becoming more religious and Belton remembered him being surprisingly aggressive and confrontational about this. He was also becoming more physical, which Belton attributed to his new friendship with a former U.S. Navy SEAL turned pro golfer, Chad Metcalf, who he had met through a golf friend of his father's. Harry was training more aggressively than usual and incorporating some SEAL-style training.

Chad, who was married and about ten years older than Harry, told me he wasn't actually training Harry—and thought some SEAL-style trainings didn't help golfers at all. But Harry had asked him a lot of questions, and Chad was aware he was pushing himself. And since "somewhere that summer he also found Jesus, and was very excited about that," their conversations, as they were getting to know each other on the golf course, included a lot of "Bible stuff" and "SEAL stuff." Nothing about it seemed out of the ordinary to Chad.

But it did to his brother. "Harry was always an athlete, and that summer he got into the best shape I ever saw him in," Belton said. "But for some reason he was really fixated on military-style workouts and the military mindset and I just thought, 'Where the hell is all this coming from?'

"Once we had some of our cousins over at the ranch and we were playing Ping-Pong and he started to shove me a little bit. So, I gave him the finger or something and he started choking me, up against the wall. I mean ankles off the floor, not good. Our cousins had to pull him off me. Afterward, one of them asked me, I think his words were, 'Is Harry losing his mind?' He was genuinely concerned."

The first signal Mark recalled came at the end of the summer, when he and his sons drove to California to take Belton to college. They drove straight from Texas to their hotel in Manhattan Beach, and after a very long day, the car was still packed with all of Belton's stuff. But Harry said he wanted to go see the famous Hollywood sign. And when Mark said that could wait until the next day, Harry insisted he wanted to see the sign "now!"

"He was acting very strangely," Mark recalled. "He wanted to take Belton's car, which was packed with everything he owned. So, he just went outside and walked around. He was a little bit psychotic about going to the Hollywood sign." Belton recalled that, later on, Harry "just stole my keys" and did take his packed-up car and drove around anyway. They later argued about it.

The next day, Ceci and Estella arrived, and they changed hotels. They moved Belton into his dorm room at USC, went out to dinner to celebrate Belton's birthday, and then drove to see the house Mark and Ceci had lived in when they were first married.

When they got back to the hotel room, "Harry started getting agitated," Mark recalled. "He started talking to me about religion. 'Tell me about your relationship with the Lord,'" he recalled Harry demanding. "'What is your religious life like?'"

Mark recalled feeling incredulous and acting a little dismissive. "Why are we talking about this right now?" he wanted to know. "It's your brother's birthday."

Then suddenly Harry "got all wound up, and he took his Bible and he threw it across the room at me," Mark recalled. "Right in front of his brother and sister and his mom. And I said, 'The way to get me to read that particular book isn't to throw it at me.' I was just mad."

Ceci and Mark separated the kids into different rooms and talked to them. Eventually everything calmed down. The rest of the trip was fun and uneventful.

Mark would later wonder if "this was a symptom." Belton was pretty sure this behavior wasn't normal but, he recalled, "none of us were thinking about it in terms of mental health, because that was not something any of us ever dealt with in our family. We were unfamiliar with it entirely. It just didn't even occur to us. I just thought, 'Whatever's going on, I just don't want to be around my brother.'"

Harry returned to Sewanee for his senior year. To some, he seemed different, but others didn't see it, and after he was gone, they wracked their brains trying to figure out why. It's possible this began with the head injury and was then exacerbated by the pressures on every college senior. It's possible something had been percolating even earlier.

"It's normal for seniors in college, male, about to graduate with a degree in American history, to wonder what you're going to do when May comes around," Mark said. "It didn't look like he'd play golf professionally. His golf had already suffered some before this. I mean, the great thing and the difficult thing about golf is, you get judged every day. And he didn't really perform as a golfer or progress very much when he was in school." He was still good, and a generous teacher to his teammates—and, when he was home, to his sister—but it looked like he was going to need to consider graduate school, or a job right out of school, and be a golf enthusiast like his father.

Mark recalled that during the fall Ceci suggested to Harry that maybe after he graduated college, he could take a year and try playing pro golf. But Mark made it clear he didn't think that was a good idea. "Sadly, in golf, you get judged by your ability every day—what did you shoot today," he said. "By that measure, pro golf didn't make sense. And the general thing I told Harry, which is true for me as well, you don't have to play golf professionally to use your golf ability to your advantage."

Harry's senior golf team picture showed he had let his hair grow a little longer. And after several years of being featured prominently in the coverage of the Sewanee golf team, he was only mentioned once the entire fall—when the team won the Piedmont College Fall Classic in Georgia. He finished twenty-ninth with a two-day total of 164.

His friend Garrett said he didn't notice anything worrisome about Harry that fall, but did recognize that he seemed "a little different," more physical than before. "He was going through this phase of 'chasing the lightning,'" he recalled. "He was really edgy, outdoorsy, thrill-seeking, full of adrenaline. He was working out heavier, wanted to do all the hiking trails and, just, seek adventure, I guess." But Garrett did also note that this was the first year he and Harry weren't rooming together, so they didn't see each other quite as often.

One incident from the fall that did stand out to everyone, however, was when Harry totaled his truck just before parents weekend. He was joy-riding off-road on one of the many beautiful wooded mountain paths near Sewanee and smashed head-on into a tree.

Harry's Navy SEAL golf friend Chad remembered getting a panicked text from him about the crash: "I wrecked my truck, what should I do?"

Chad texted back, "did you call your dad?"

And Harry texted, "no, I'm scared to."

Chad insisted Harry call Mark, which he finally did. But Harry didn't tell his father the whole story. First, he claimed he was alone in the truck. It was only days later, after his friends were talking about the crash during parents weekend, that he admitted other details to Mark, including that there had been a young woman in the car, and she had been hurt. She had apparently hit her head and had a concussion, and because they were out of cell phone range, Harry had to carry her almost a mile until they could find help.

Harry said that his airbag had deployed, and he had not hit his head or been hurt, but Mark noticed a large bruise on his arm. And nobody thought to explore if the crash had further affected his brain in any way—which can happen regardless of actual impact if the head is whipped forward. While some in sports medicine and military medicine were paying attention to issues concerning traumatic brain injuries and the impacts of secondary insults to the brain, that was not on anyone's radar for something like a crash from which Harry walked away almost without a scratch.

After parents weekend, Harry and Garrett were in the home stretch of finishing the thirty-page paper required for history majors. "Harry's paper was on the psychology of the Marines," he recalled. "He was interested in how they stuck it out through thick and thin, and the camaraderie of being an American hero."

The two spent a lot of time together in the library, all pretty normal except for one late fall afternoon when Harry left early, saying he wanted to do a trail run. At around 4:30 P.M., he called Garrett and said he was in trouble. He had been standing on a seven-foot-tall rock trying to set up to take a picture of the sunset from Perimeter Trail, when he slipped. "I fell," he told Garrett, "and now I'm afraid to move. Can you come get me?" Garrett drove the half hour there and then followed the trail in the cold and fading light to where Harry was waiting.

"By this time, he was up and fine," Garrett recalled. "He was downplaying the whole thing. He was, like, 'I kinda fell.' I asked if he was okay, and all he said was 'So where should we have dinner?' He walked away from it and was normal after that. But it was a little weird at the time."

They were back at the library the next day, just like normal, and soon turned in their papers and went home for Thanksgiving break.

While Garrett wasn't worried about any changes in his friend, Harry's brother, Belton, was. When Harry came to pick Belton up at the airport in San Antonio, he was "clearly depressed. He just looked like a sad sack, clearly having a lot of really melancholy thoughts. At the time, honestly, I was happy to see my brother and thought, 'Oh great, he's not mean anymore.' He was nicer. But, of course, that's another personality shift right there, and it should have been very obvious to more well-trained eyes."

He remembered their conversation during the ninety-minute drive to Fredericksburg vividly: "Harry was gazing open-eyed at the horizon, asking big questions in a melancholy way," he recalled. "It was starkly different than how he had been during the summer. I had never heard him ask these kinds of questions before. I don't remember the words he was using, I remember more the tone, and also that the questions were a bit more moral in nature, questions about what was right and wrong."

I asked, did it seem like something spiritual in nature, or was he asking if he was partying too much, something like that?

"I think it was more of, y'know, 'Am I doing things right here?' And I was a freshman in college. I wasn't really able to process that kind of questioning."

Did he seem afraid he had done something wrong?

"Maybe so," Belton said. "I don't know what he did in college. I mean, he slept around, partied a lot. Maybe that weighed heavily on him. I do think there was a lot that he didn't tell us. And I think my mom and dad noted there were a lot of discrepancies between what Harry had told them and what his friends then told them. Also, some of his friends at college seemed unwilling to come forward about what happened with Harry at school. But I don't know if it was, 'We can't tell them about what happened,' or maybe they were just uncomfortable talking to my parents in that situation.

"A big part of my grieving process has been the accepting that I'm not going to get the answers."

Harry returned to school after Thanksgiving and remained until the fall semester ended. During Christmas break, there were parties that the family always attended, all in San Antonio. Belton remembered that Harry "started to become antisocial. He would come, dance a little, but then he would usually excuse himself early, and you couldn't get him to come back out of the hotel room.

"I remember one big party, tuxedos and everything, just a massive ordeal, very close friends of ours. . . . There's, like, a thousand people at this party. And Harry just went in early, and we had to go try to bring him out, telling him, 'People want to talk to you.'

"It was clear he had a cloud over his head. At that point, other people—you know, friends and family—were asking, 'What's wrong with Harry?'"

The idea that any of this could have something to do with his head injury "just didn't occur to me," Belton said. "But I was worried about my brother, and I do remember thinking, 'Is this what, you know, heading toward depression and suicide looks like?' I just didn't know enough to understand what I was looking at. So, I didn't want to bring it up with anybody. Frankly, that's a huge factor of my guilt in hindsight is that I didn't bring it up because I was scared to bring it up. I mean, I can't speak for anybody else. But I remember very clearly thinking, 'If he is, I'm afraid. And if he isn't, I'm afraid that bringing it up is going to give him the idea or is going to have some sort of negative repercussion.'"

He noted, "There was no history of how to handle something like that in our family; both sides of our family had severe alcoholics, and that's what we worried about. And I did notice that Harry cut back on drinking during the holidays. He had, at most, one or two drinks."

Classes at Sewanee began again on January 16. His college friend Garrett hadn't heard much from Harry over break, which seemed unusual—he had sent Harry a few texts but got no responses. Garrett was feeling the last-semester pressure, not knowing what to do after college. He knew Harry was feeling it, too.

"He was off," he recalled. "He was trying to make himself better, but I think he was just pushing himself way too hard, taking himself way too seriously." He also wasn't playing or practicing golf very much. And, with his workouts cut back, he had put on some weight.

About a month into the semester, Harry called Garrett out of the blue.

"Hey, man," he said, "can you come meet me at Hodgson?" It was one of the dorms, and Garrett drove there "thinking everything is gravy, I'm gonna graduate in a matter of weeks with my best friend, Harry. But when I got there, he was coming back from his storage unit, which I thought was a little odd."

Harry walked up to him and said, "I'm going home." He was quitting school.

"We have six fucking weeks left of college," Garrett shot back, "and I am not getting that diploma without you right behind me."

But Harry was sure. "I gotta do this. I don't feel right," Garrett recalled him saying. "Dad's gonna get some kind of specialist. I have to go. I need help. I won't make it if I stay."

Garrett, stunned, pleaded with him, offering the only thing he could think of. "I will . . . quit drinking right now for the rest of the year if you stay here with me," he recalled saying. "And, last semester senior year, that would be asking a lot." But Harry's mind was made up.

Garrett suggested doctors and counselors he could call on campus or in nearby Nashville at Vanderbilt. "I just kept saying, 'Please don't do this,' but he had made up his mind," Garrett told me. "And this is such a huge regret of mine, that I didn't try harder to get him to stay. I was unfamiliar with mental illness. Not saying I haven't had my fair share of breakdowns and just kind of being overwhelmed by stuff. I've experienced a few panic attacks, but nothing as serious as the rabbit hole of depression. So, I finally just told him, 'Okay, Harry, you're gonna go get help, you'll get better, and you'll be back in a few weeks.'"

The way Garrett recalled it, "he didn't say the word *depressed;* he didn't say the word *suicidal;* he didn't say anything scary like that. But what he said was scary."

They were standing in Harry's room, and Garrett didn't know what else to say.

"I finally just said, 'I love you. Take care of yourself. Please get help.' And he said, 'I know I need help.' And that was the A-bomb that was dropped on me that day."

As Garrett left, Harry headed out of his room, got into his already-packed black four-door pickup truck, and drove away. Garrett immediately called his parents in Montgomery. His father called Mark, who he knew from parents weekend; he said he was violating his son's confidence by reaching out, but he it thought was important.

But Mark already knew. He had the same conversation with Harry a couple of hours earlier. "Harry told me, 'I can't stay here another day.' He sounded terrible, like he was distraught; his voice was not his voice. The whole thing was so out of character. I finally just said, 'What would you like me to do?' And he just said, 'I'm leaving here.' Although he didn't say it to me directly, I did think there was a danger of suicide. He said he was packing and he was going to drive home. I told him not to do that."

He spoke to Ceci, and they agreed Mark should fly to Tennessee and drive home with Harry. They agreed to meet at the Nashville airport and make the twelve-hour drive home together.

When Mark saw his son, he looked different. He was heavier. "He had gained maybe twenty-five pounds." Mark discovered Harry had stopped practicing golf. The spring season was scheduled to begin the next week, the Reeder Cup at Lookout Mountain, Georgia, and Harry apparently had no interest in playing.

"We drove straight through," Mark recalled, "and I tried as best I could to draw him out. When I got to Nashville, I offered to drive. He said he wanted to. I wasn't worried about him, you know, running us into a tree. I wasn't thinking of that. I just thought it would be easier for him to talk if I drove."

Mark asked some questions but made it clear he wasn't trying to pressure Harry. "There are no right or wrong answers to these questions," he said. "I'm just trying to understand and see if I can help." He told Harry he didn't care if he returned to school and finished the semester. He didn't care about anything but his son's health.

Before leaving for Nashville, Mark had called a psychiatrist he knew, who he had seen for individual therapy and a few sessions of couples therapy before he and Ceci split. The psychiatrist told Mark, "Don't let him out of your sight" and requested that Harry be brought directly to his office for an evaluation.

After twelve hours on the road, stopping only to pee and eat, they arrived in Austin and went straight to the psychiatrist's office. Harry was in with him for nearly two hours, after which he came out and, as Mark remembered it, the doctor told him it was okay for Harry to go home, and he could continue treating him as an outpatient. He wanted to see Harry again in a few days and didn't view the risk of self-harm high enough to warrant hospitalization.

"I recall him saying, 'We need a little more time with him, but he's okay,'" Mark said. "I don't remember if he put him on medication straightaway. I think he just wanted him to be away from school for a few days and then come back, which is what happened. He suggested it might just be a 'situational depression' that could improve now that he was away from whatever might have been bothering him at school."

When he got back to the ranch, his mother also suggested he get faith-based counseling.

"To be honest, I didn't see the point of faith-based therapy," Mark said. "I didn't think it would do any harm, but you're not going to pray your way out of a situation like this, as far as I'm concerned. I told Ceci that. And let's just say we disagreed."

Belton understood his parents' disagreement. "I think my mom has a large degree of skepticism toward mental health just because of the pharmaceutical industry," he said. "She's inherently distrustful of that, as many people are very well within their rights to be. As am I, honestly. And I don't think she trusts the nature of pharmaceuticals as an approach to mental health.

"So, there was a fork in the road between the way our parents perceived as the right way to approach this."

Harry's younger sister, Estella, then a sophomore in high school, recalled in an online interview being thrilled to have her big brother and golf buddy home unexpectedly, but she was also a little confused. On one of his first nights home, they were lying in her bed together watching a golf documentary, and they were just chatting until she finally had to ask, "Why are you home—I'm so happy you're home, but what happened?"

He told her, "If I had stayed there, in Tennessee at school, I wouldn't be here right now. And I couldn't do that to you."

She didn't quite understand what he was saying. "'What do you mean you wouldn't be here?'" she recalled asking. "And I didn't really ask any questions, I was just like, 'Okay, well great,' and I gave him a hug and we didn't talk about it anymore."

She didn't tell her parents about the conversation but later wished she had. And they didn't tell her that Harry had already said basically the same thing to them.

HARRY WAS HOME for the next two months, and the immediate danger seemed to pass. He didn't look well, and he was obviously depressed and struggling. Nobody around him felt he was at risk for self-harm—or, at least, nobody treating him shared anything with the family that suggested they were worried.

But mostly Mark found himself frustrated when the psychiatrist in Austin wouldn't share any details of Harry's condition or treatment.

"I called him and said, 'What do I need to know?'" Mark recalled. "And he said, 'Well, this is a little frustrating but I can't really talk to you about Harry. He's twenty-two years old, it's between me and him.' And I said, 'Well, that doesn't help me very much, other than the fact that you're telling me he's okay.'"

He thought the situation was absurd—as do many parents and family members who cannot get information about relatives they are caring for—but he figured that if the doctor said he didn't need to be overly concerned, he could be patient. He and Ceci did find out that the psychiatrist, after seeing Harry again several days after the first session, had ruled out "situational depression" and diagnosed Harry with "clinical depression" (or what is usually called "major depressive disorder"). They also knew he was prescribed medication, but Mark didn't recall knowing what it was. He told me he recently contacted the psychiatrist for the first time in six years and learned that Harry was taking 20 mg of the antidepressant and antianxiety medicine escitalopram (Lexapro). It is unclear how seriously Harry took the recommendation not to drink alcohol while taking this medication; it can worsen depression and increase suicide risk.

The most surprising thing about Harry was that he seemed to have lost almost all interest in golf. He rarely played or practiced—when he did, it was only to help his sister—and he was no longer getting up in the morning and working out. In fact, some mornings he wasn't getting up at all.

In early March, Mark tried to convince Harry to come into Austin for the annual South by Southwest music and arts festival. Harry had always loved SXSW in the past. This time he came to Austin but didn't leave Mark's house. He expressed concern about a big family wedding upcoming in San Antonio, and he worried how he would explain to people why he had left school. He was embarrassed: "What am I going to tell them?"

Mark tried to make it clear to him, "It's not unusual for anyone to take time off from school in this or any other family. Tell them you're taking a break. Nobody cares. If they ask why, just ignore them."

His once fearless son was now mortified at the prospect of being judged.

Before Harry had to go back to Fredericksburg, the two of them had a little more time together. Mark was sitting on his couch; Harry was in a chair nearby, in blue jeans, a white shirt, and a sweater.

"Why don't we go out and walk around SXSW?" Mark asked.

"Why don't we just sit here and talk?" Harry replied.

Mark thought this might be the moment when his son would really confide in him. Instead, "Harry just looked out the window and said, 'I just don't know.' Then he said it again, 'I just don't know.'

And that was scary to me. And when I asked him what he meant, he kept saying, 'I just don't know. I just don't know,' still looking out the window."

This was, Mark told me, the only time he was worried about whether he should let Harry drive more than an hour back to Fredericksburg. But he did, and everything was fine.

On March 24, Harry turned twenty-two. The next day the whole family was in San Antonio for a big family wedding, which Harry did attend and seemed to enjoy.

Belton remembered seeing his brother at the wedding for the first time in over two months. Harry was heavier. "He let himself go a little bit physically," he remembered. "He wasn't fat, but you could tell he wasn't exercising." But he didn't seem as sad to Belton as he did before. "It's easy to think in hindsight," he said, "that since he took his own life soon after that, he was, and I'm trying to find the right words for it, not so much saying goodbye to people, but he seemed peaceable, he was being nice to everybody. He just didn't have any more of that negativity or aggression in him.

"I think we thought, 'Maybe we're getting somewhere because he's not as bad as he was during Christmastime.' I don't know. Maybe it's because he knew that this was the last time we were going to see each other. I just don't know."

The last time Belton saw him was when Harry dropped him off at the airport after the wedding. "There was no grand final communication with me," Belton said. "He very kindly said 'Bye' and 'Have fun the rest of your semester . . . don't do anything silly.'"

THE NEXT WEEKEND was the Masters Tournament, the Super Bowl of golf (and something the McMurrey family cared about much more than the Super Bowl). Mark called Harry and begged him to come to Austin for the weekend and attend a big Masters watching party he had always enjoyed in the past.

"He told me, 'I just want to be by myself,'" Mark remembered.

On Masters Saturday, Mark went to Fredericksburg and played nine holes of golf with Estella, who was preparing for the state high school tournament. They asked Harry to play, but much to their frustration, he said no.

On Sunday, April 9, the final day of the Masters, Harry and Estella watched the tournament together at home. Like everyone else, they were amazed that Sergio Garcia—a Spanish golfer who had recently started spending more time in Austin—was still in contention. While Garcia had been a phenom as a young player, at age thirty-seven he was now viewed as having missed his chance to ever win golf's top tournament.

At 7:53 P.M., the Masters ended after a sudden death playoff. Garcia had won.

Harry immediately texted his dad two words, "El Toro!" meaning "tough as a bull."

Mark texted him right back, "Just like you . . . El Toro!" It was their last communication.

Sometime later that evening, Harry Bennett McMurrey left his upstairs bedroom and quietly exited the house. He walked the hundred yards to the barn and then around it, to an Airstream trailer that was parked there, sometimes used as a guest room. That's where he took his life.

The exact time of death was not known but was estimated to be about 5:30 A.M. Mark assumed that was right, because that was when, lying very soundly asleep in his bed in Austin, he suddenly sprang straight up for no reason.

"I don't know what it was," he said. "But if you believe in a universal life force, it might have been when he took his life."

He looked at the clock and went back to sleep. It was several hours before Ceci called with the horrible news.

Estella found out at school—she was called out of a morning class and told her mom was there for her, which made no sense to her until she saw Ceci's tear-stained face. Belton recalled getting the call from Estella that woke him out of a sound sleep. He had been up working on his student film until 2:00 A.M. and generally had been so involved with the project over the previous weeks that he hadn't been in touch with home very much.

"I knew before I picked up the phone why she was calling," he said. "And I remember thinking, 'Great, this is what I get for being too scared to speak up.' Like, the one thing I was exactly afraid of, and too afraid to bring it up with him or anybody, is what happened. I mean, that's not *why* it happened, because I didn't bring it up. But I just remember being nineteen years old and feeling guilty about it."

He thought for a second. "I guess in a way," he said, "a part of me will always be nineteen years old because I'll never get to see my big brother older. In some way I'll be permanently stunted, the same way that sometimes I feel I've been stunted in my understanding of relationships because of my parents splitting up when I was younger. A part of you just gets stuck at this moment in time at this age."

Mark wasn't told much that would help him understand.

"Harry left a note," he said, "It was in his bedroom, but the police took it, so I didn't see it. And when they gave it back, I already knew what it said. But I didn't want to see it, and I still don't. I'm a very visual person, and if I see it, that image is going to be stuck in my brain. And I'd rather not have it there."

What is stuck in his brain are memories from later that evening, when he decided he needed to stay over in Harry's bedroom. He remembered the five wide-open copies of the New Testament, which Harry had lined up on his long skinny desk by the window, each one with handwritten notes in the margins. He remembered the empty beer cans, which he assumed Harry had finished before going to the Airstream. He remembered picking up pieces of Harry's dirty clothes and bringing them to his nose because they still smelled like his son. He remembered putting on one of Harry's favorite guayaberas—a multicolored Cuban short-sleeve shirt with his initials on it—and a pair of his tan hiking shorts. And then he got into Harry's unmade bed and sobbed until he fell asleep.

"You just wanna be as close to them as you can," he told me. "That's all you have, right? You have his clothes, his smell."

IT HAS BEEN over six years since Harry died. His memory is strong among his family and friends—when I talked to his college roommate Garrett, at a certain point he started crying and couldn't stop. But Harry's legacy, and the lessons of his suicide, are just beginning to be processed. I am deeply proud of my cousins Mark and Belton for agreeing to talk to me about this, no matter how painful the experience. It gets us closer to exploring the varying narratives of how this could have happened and, as Mark's friend suggested, trying to get past the *whys*. It also just seems to help to talk about it, even if the conversations don't end neatly.

I told Mark about the surprising recent research about suicides, showing that while a great many of them are the end result of untreated or undertreated mental illness—and underutilized prevention techniques—there are new ways of thinking about the different ways a brain can get to thinking about self-harm. I've met researchers who explain there can be something like an A-fib for the brain, where there is some circuit breaker that isn't working because of, say, a traumatic brain injury. And there can be very temporary impulsivity without mental or brain disease.

These ideas are intriguing, interesting approaches to scientific and psychological research. They are also concepts that parents discuss and mull over after losing a child to suicide. But we have to be careful not to debate them when someone living says they don't want to be alive anymore.

And that is a big part of the challenge, especially when, like me, you live and work simultaneously both in the world of treatment of illness and prevention of self-harm and in the world of bereavement care for those, like my cousin, who have already suffered the ultimate loss.

One day when we were discussing this, Mark was going through what he wished he and his family and their doctors and counselors had done better or differently to keep Harry alive—more aggressive brain injury care, more aggressive psychiatric care, hospitalization, *something*. Then he noted that he had a friend who had just lost a fifteen-year-old daughter to suicide, after she was treated in and out of hospitals for fourteen months. He said the lesson they took from this was, "It's almost impossible to stop somebody from taking their own life if they really want to."

In that moment I could understand how the idea of inevitability might bring Mark comfort, and I've had that feeling myself when I've lost friends and family members to suicide.

But part of me wondered how to also help Mark feel comforted by the fact that, increasingly, we do have ways of preventing some suicides, and proof those techniques—short-term talk therapies, medicines, emergency room procedures, apps—really can work.

I keep thinking about what Mark said to Harry's doctor. We

absolutely do need a "bigger radar screen" when it comes to any kind of suicidal thoughts. And we need much more education and uniformity of response for every time that radar picks up a ping.

AT THE END of one of our sessions, Mark told me a story about a visit he made to the Cape not long after Harry's death. Mark went sailing with the family, on my dad's old boat, the *Mya,* with a group that included our beloved aunt, Ethel Kennedy, who is well into her nineties.

"Patrick, you know, if you've never been on that boat, it's hard to describe how intimate it is behind the wheel," he said, as I nodded. "So, Ethel and I are squeezed in back there. We're practically on top of each other we're squeezed so close. And we have to hold on to each other every time we're coming about—we're not switching sides since Ethel is not going to move. You understand what I'm saying, right?

"This is a couple of months after Harry died, and we got to talking about grief. And there's probably not a better person to talk to about grief than Ethel. And she says to me, 'How are you doing?' And I say, 'Well, I'm not very happy with God right now,' because Ethel knew Harry enough to know what an incredible person he was. And I said, 'I don't understand why God wanted this one back. So, I'm not real happy with God right now.'"

She looked up at Mark from their scrunched-in position, and she said, "You just have to have faith. And the sooner you can get to where you're able to rely on your faith, the better off you're going to be. I'm not saying it's going to happen immediately, but you need to get there."

I had to ask, because I've had these conversations with my aunt as well: Did that resonate with you? Does faith help you?

"I still struggle with that," he said. "Because I just don't understand. I mean, there's obviously some bigger stuff going on. You would have to believe pretty strongly that this series of circumstances is somehow connected to a bigger story that's beyond our understanding. It's the kind of suspension of disbelief which becomes belief. So, you have to believe that this is somehow all tied together. I'm not there yet."

BELTON HAD ONE more story he wanted to share about his brother and anniversaries, which I know are times that deeply challenge all families who have lost a member to suicide. Harry's birthday was in late March, and he died less than three weeks later, so that period is always tough. But in 2021, all the feelings and the "big grappling questions" came back again in an even bigger way because Belton had recently turned twenty-three, but it wasn't until the anniversary came around again that he realized he was "older than Harry will ever be."

He was particularly far from home—in fact, he had been far from home a lot since Harry died, especially after finishing at USC. He was doing research for a film project in Central Africa, in the rainforest of Okapi Wildlife Preserve in the Ituri Province of Eastern Democratic Republic of the Congo.

"I was in the middle of a ridiculously dangerous place in the Congo," he told me. "In a way it was a nice place to be because all the people I was dealing with had lost somebody. In fact, in that part of the world, everybody has lost somebody, often in ways that are horrific beyond description."

Belton was feeling "gloomy that day" and some of the people he was with noticed and asked why. He explained—in Swahili, which he was still learning—that his older brother had died. He told them Harry had taken his own life, and he still had a lot of unanswered questions about it.

"And they looked at me," he recalled, "and the word for a white person in Swahili is '*mzungu*,' and they puzzled for a second that a *mzungu* could suffer a tragedy like ones they had suffered—situations where 'we've loved someone and we will never get any answers to our questions about why this happened.'"

He was initially surprised they were interested at all. "I was expecting their reaction to be, like, 'Get over it, welcome to Congo,'" he told me. "We were in a place that has been war-torn for several generations, exploited for hundreds of years. But then they started asking questions, and I tried to explain—and since I was working on my Swahili, I was using very simple terms. And they asked if I had pictures, so I was showing them pictures on my phone of our ranch, and how fat our cattle are, and just how green our grass is, and, you know, our cute little dogs . . ."

Belton recalled how "incredulous they were that this could happen in America, that someone could be so unhappy, in a place they perceived as perfect, that they would take their own life. I tried to explain to them that my brother had, you know, difficulties mentally. These were people who experience things that humans should never have to see or go through or have done to them. And I was just very touched by their empathy. I learned a lot from them about different dimensions of grief. And how you just have to carry on."

Chapter Eight

Bob

In the summer of 1986, Bob Kazel had to start lying again.

After graduating top of his class from one of the country's best undergraduate journalism programs—the Medill School at Northwestern, just outside his hometown of Chicago—he was twenty-two years old and the envy of his very competitive peers. The tall, lanky guy with cropped curly hair and a nerdy disposition had scored one of the best first jobs possible: a paid internship at the *Miami Herald,* at a time when Florida newspapers were considered the stepping stones to dream jobs in the biggest newspaper towns.

All Bob had to do was fly to Florida—where he had already done two summer internships—and claim his position at the *Herald*. But he couldn't. And he didn't want to tell the paper, or anyone else, the reason why.

Bob had taken five years to finish Northwestern. He had left during his first semester and, technically, moved back to his Chicago home with his mom—who had been raising him and his brother alone since her husband died when Bob was fourteen. But, in fact, much of his time away from school had been spent not far from campus, in the inpatient psychiatric ward at Evanston Hospital, where he was treated for what was then called manic-depressive illness (now bipolar disorder). He had responded so well to the only medicine available at the time, lithium, that he was able to start school over, enjoying four years of good health and great reporting and writing, and summer newspaper internships in Chicago and Florida, including one at the *Herald,* which wanted him back. And he desperately wanted to go.

He tried to buy some time by claiming he was having "health problems." When pressed, he described them as "stomach troubles" for which he needed "more tests."

He couldn't tell them he was in a psychiatric hospital. Again.

So, he kept asking his editor for just a little more time, allowing his health situation to resolve before starting work. Eventually the paper couldn't wait any longer and gave the job to someone else—never knowing why their young prospect never showed up.

But while Bob couldn't tell them, he did decide to confide in one person besides his mother and brother. It was Jonathan Eig, a driven, bighearted New Yorker who had succeeded at Medill as a breaking news reporter just as Bob had excelled in features. The two "Medill-dos" (as some Northwestern journalists call each other) had remained in touch by mail after graduation—partly out of mutual admiration, partly to keep track of each other in the career climb. Jon was at *The San Jose Mercury News* and didn't know what to make of Bob's gastrointestinal excuses for delaying Miami.

Finally, on July 23, 1986, Bob sent him a five-page handwritten letter, in which he admitted, "The truth is I've been bullshitting you about why I'm here. . . . The bald truth, Jonathan, is that I'm at the tail end of a 2½-week stay in Evanston Hospital's intensive-care psych ward. . . . I'm a manic-depressive. I don't know your knowledge of that. You might be summoning up images . . . of knife-wielding lunatics who steal babies or eat them, or worse. But you're more hip certainly . . . so I can't imagine you're being freaked out by a concept like mental illness. I imagine you might be intrigued, actually."

With that letter began a friendship that has lasted forty years. It has spanned the maddening cycles of Bob's illness—which have broken through every four or five years like tortured clockwork. After each recurrence, he has managed to rebuild a slightly different life, first as a successful reporter at the New Orleans *Times-Picayune,* then returning to Chicago where he worked at several smaller publications and trade journals. And then years doing writing, teaching, and meaningful volunteerism—in journalism, as well as in the mental health and LGBTQ+ communities doing peer support. (After years of what he jokingly refers to as being "double closeted," Bob came out as being gay.)

Jon ended up moving back to Chicago as well. And as Bob's health cycled and got worse, he became more a part of Jon's family, joining him and his wife, Jennifer, for holiday meals and acting as a loving "uncle" to the Eigs' three children. After Bob's mom died in 2001, Jon got more of the manic phone calls—from Bob and, occasionally, the police. But their friendship endures. (Jon is now a bestselling author of big biographies and is friends with my co-author, which is how I met him and Bob.)

The story of how Bob Kazel has lived a life requiring him to constantly reevaluate and adjust to accommodate his progressing mental illness is really moving to me. Today, at age sixty, Bob is suffering some consequences of the early high dosing of lithium. He is on dialysis three times a week and now lives in a nursing home with a dialysis unit. He is there also because the facility will accept his Social Security Disability Insurance, Medicaid, and other government support.

The other consequence of his illness is that he hasn't been able to earn a living for years and has long since spent all his savings paying for care. He continues doing some teaching and writing (and chatting with friends) from his room.

As he wrote to Jon in that very first letter: "Don't let my saga get you down. That's not how I feel; it's not how you should feel. Manic depression has been a fascinating condition . . . that has taught me a lot and shown me lots of sides of my personality and potential. In many ways, I feel lucky. In many ways I feel crummy, especially when my life gets thrown out of order. But life doesn't come with any guarantees, right?"

BOB'S EARLIEST MEMORIES of mental illness in his family are things that, at the time, nobody talked about. Bob grew up in the North Park section of Chicago. As a child, he didn't see his paternal grandmother often. But he told me that when she came for family events, "she was always crying. Like, out of control. I don't remember any time that I ever saw her when she wasn't crying. It was rumored that she had spent time in mental hospitals, but I really had no idea what to think of this, and it wasn't really spoken about."

He said his father, Sidney, was never diagnosed with bipolar disorder, "but retrospectively," Bob said, "I can see signs." Sidney was an electrical engineer for a research institute that did a lot of work for the U.S. Air Force—but, deep in his heart, "he was an inventor, a very brilliant inventor." When Bob was in grade school, his father quit his job and started his own company in the family basement. He invented several devices that he patented but eventually returned to his research job.

He would also "get into these moods where he would 'disappear' for weeks or months at a time. In our house we had what we called our 'den,' a spare bedroom that had been converted into a rec room but also had a bed. He would just withdraw into himself there, and not communicate with the rest of the family." His father would eat and sleep in that den, and Bob didn't know what to make of it. His father "never saw a psychiatrist, because he was against psychiatry, thought it was a waste of money."

When Bob was fourteen, his father died in a single-car accident on a Chicago expressway while driving to work. He crashed into one of the pillars holding up an overpass. "Police didn't offer any explanation for what happened," he recalled. "They said he might have swerved to avoid another car. But it was never really explained."

And when Bob eventually became ill, he said his mother, Beverly, never suggested it was something he might have inherited from his father. "She blamed herself," he said. "She thought maybe she had put too much pressure on me academically." It was a time when psychoanalytic theory was still focused primarily on blaming mothers and mothering for everything.

Bob always wanted to go to Northwestern, located just north of Chicago in Evanston, and become a journalist. The summer after his junior year of high school, he studied there through the Medill Cherub program. And after his senior year, he spent the summer as a copy boy at the *Chicago Sun-Times,* home of the legendary columnist Mike Royko, who Bob idolized.

At Northwestern, he was able to get a coveted single dorm room as a freshman. He gave no thought, initially, to the fact that it was in the Foster-Walker Complex—a dorm of all singles, which was referred to by some as "Suicide Hall" because of the surprising number of attempted and completed suicides by its residents. Foster-Walker had recently been featured in a local PBS documentary called *College Can Be Killing.*

He started school "feeling good, feeling challenged," he said. "But then, really quickly, I started feeling overwhelmed. I was suddenly very uncertain about myself. I had this irrational fear that I was gonna flunk out of school—even though my grades were great—and have to go to a much less selective school. I kept thinking maybe I wasn't cut out for Northwestern after all."

Increasingly anxious and unable to sleep, he started getting talk therapy from a social worker through the student health service. "I began getting these strange psychosomatic symptoms, a feeling that my life was in danger and I had some terrible disease," he recalled. "I was constantly pacing around, nervous all the time."

He was referred to a psychiatrist, with an office just a few blocks off campus. "He didn't help me very much," he said, "although I didn't tell him very much. Mostly at those sessions I just sat there in silence with him. He stared at me, and I was extremely depressed." Before the semester ended, he withdrew from school and, with the help of his psychiatrist, was voluntarily admitted to the University's Evanston Hospital in the psychiatric ward.

"Back then, the same psychiatrist who had been treating me could come see me in the hospital," he recalled. "I saw him every day for forty minutes. Which is unheard of today when you might see a hospitalist psychiatrist for five minutes if you're lucky." (Most hospitals, not just mental health hospitals, now have a salaried in-house staff of physicians called "hospitalists" who take care of inpatients instead of your outpatient treatment professionals.)

Bob recalled being diagnosed first, incorrectly it turned out, with schizophrenia. A lot of people were still being diagnosed incorrectly with schizophrenia then, because without many useful treatments, it was challenging to tell diagnoses apart. (Psychiatric diagnosis was also still developing in the 1980s; the first edition of the *DSM* that offered truly medical diagnostic guidance, *DSM-3,* was published in 1980 and updated in 1987, taking a while to catch on in a mental health world still dominated by psychoanalytic ideas.) Bob was treated with a succession of early antipsychotics: trifluoperazine (Stelazine), haloperidol (Haldol), and fluphenazine (Prolixin). He recalled spending "ninety-seven percent of my time in bed, just lying there miserable." His happiest memory of the long inpatient stay was his mother, visiting him at the hospital twice a day, always arriving with a Baskin-Robbins milkshake to make up for the bad food. She also sometimes brought her amazing homemade chocolate chip mandel bread.

He hated the way the drugs made him feel. "I felt like a zombie," he said, "like I was separated from my true thoughts and I couldn't connect with them. It was very disturbing." He left the hospital on the antipsychotic medications but soon told his mother he needed to stop taking them. Within a month, he no longer felt depressed at all—because he was having his first-ever manic experience.

Manic reactions begin with hypomania, a mild exuberance that makes people feel creative, empowered, hypervigilant, even euphoric, the mind suddenly making smart, surprising connections.

It's fun while it lasts, but it never lasts. I can tell you from personal experience. And I have a much milder form of the illness than Bob does.

During his mania, Bob convinced a local businessman to invest $2,000 in an idea he had concerning personal computers—which very few people had in the early '80s—and how they might be connected. He imagined an early form of email that you would only be able to receive at a public place like a terminal in a McDonald's. He imagined newspapers being delivered over the computer. But he was also eighteen, and manic, and had no idea how to run a company or make these things actually happen.

Soon he needed to be hospitalized again. This time he was properly diagnosed, and correctly treated with mental health's most recent wonder drug—lithium.

He had read about the treatment in *Moodswing: The Third Revolution in Psychiatry,* a popular book from the 1970s that described how mental health diagnosis had been transformed first by drugs that helped dampen psychotic symptoms, then by drugs that helped dampen depressive mood symptoms—allowing clinicians and patients to better understand the differences between the symptoms—and then by lithium, approved by the FDA in 1970, which dampened the severe swinging of moods from mania to depression. The success of the drugs also reinforced the idea that mental illnesses were not just psychological and triggered by life events and traumas, but also biochemical and genetic in nature. (We now know there are, besides two severities of the illness—bipolar I and II—a variety of what are called "mixed states" and that some people have "rapid cycling" between mania and depression. Classic, lithium-responding bipolar I patients like Bob often have longer, broader swings in mood.)

Bob's second hospitalization was much shorter because he responded quickly to lithium, so much so that he was able to return to college in the fall of 1982 as if nothing had happened. His only major concession to his illness—although, over the years, the illness has required many other concessions—was his decision to live at home in North Park, not on Northwestern's campus.

Because he lived at home, his colleagues at the paper only got to know him so well—he was at the office for all the writing and editing, but not involved in the socializing once the paper was put to bed. This kept him at arm's length from some of his colleagues socially, but it didn't keep his star from rising at the paper. His first job at *The Daily Northwestern* was in the "off-campus bureau," but he later covered the city politics beat, including Evanston city council. He was able to sail through Northwestern with excellent grades, clips from *The Daily Northwestern*—not just smart reporting but elegant feature writing—and impressive internships every summer, at *The Chicago Reporter,* the *Fort Lauderdale Sun Sentinel,* and the *Miami Herald.*

By his senior year, he was arguably the strongest writing voice at the paper, not only covering his beat but writing other inspiring pieces. The day in January 1986 when the NASA rocket *Challenger* exploded, he was riding home from school on the Ravenswood El, watching people on the train going through the first couple of stages of profound national grief, with all the sounds of their silence. He watched them carefully, scribbled notes, and as soon as he reached his station, turned around, took the train back to campus, and wrote a memorable column capturing the moment: "Television, a keeper of dreams that had guided them all their lives around the world's realness, had betrayed their trust and shown them their own nightmares. A glimpse of chaos, of a baffling arbitrariness that they now saw clearly and would try to work out, by themselves."

THE ONE SOCIAL thing Bob did on campus was attend monthly meetings of what was called "The Lithium Clinic," a group of fellow patients with manic depression who got together at the hospital to talk about their experiences on the medication. This gave him an early appreciation for the power of peer support—on top of any personal or group therapy. It also helped him later understand how inconsistent peer support really was.

If you lived in a place like a university campus where something like this was facilitated, you might assume there were such groups everywhere, as their value was so obvious. But as he grew older and worked in different places, he came to realize just how special and rare his group, and groups like it, really were. It existed in part because it was Chicago, where the first major support group for bipolar disorder, originally called Manic Depressive Association—MDA—was founded. (MDA later grew into the national organization now called Depression and Bipolar Support Alliance, or DBSA.)

But a consistent problem nationwide was that while such peer support groups can be incredibly important to patients—in mental health and recovery groups for addiction—they could also be challenging to hold together over long periods. Like any volunteer organization, they relied on a core group of people to remain committed to each other—sometimes regardless of their own health and circumstances—and an influx of new people when regulars left.

I was, for example, incredibly fortunate that when I got sober in 2011, while living at my then girlfriend (and now wife) Amy's parents' house, there was a strong, church-based twelve-step group very close by in Absecon, New Jersey, which was there for me. And over a decade later, it remains there for me. But not everyone is that geographically lucky and most people, when they first need a group like this, are not yet well enough to find or travel to one, let alone start one.

Also, the local groups, like the local houses of worship where they sometimes meet, often have different perspectives on key issues. They can differ on whether members of the group are allowed to tell others about it (hard-core AA twelve-step is completely confidential; more liberal groups are okay with sharing). They can differ on whether members are encouraged to or discouraged from taking medication. They can differ on how religious the language in meetings will be. And sometimes the age and experience differences in members can be an issue—especially for younger people walking into a group of older, hard-seasoned vets.

But Bob was lucky to have the Lithium Clinic group available to him in college with fellow university people in it. Many people at that time weren't so fortunate, although the good news is that campus mental health and addiction support groups are much more available now.

When Bob got sick again, just after graduating from college, there was no easily identifiable reason why. Sometimes when people with mental illnesses have been doing well for an extended period, they try reducing or not taking their medication, either of which can contribute to a relapse. But Bob hadn't done anything like that. He took his meds; he saw his therapist. The only real change in his life was that he had temporarily moved onto campus because he'd been hired to help run the same Medill Cherubs summer program he had once attended. That involved some new stress, but he still didn't see the relapse coming.

After he wrote to Jon about his diagnosis, his friend had a lot of questions about the illness and the relapses, and Bob did his best to explain.

"The medication doesn't manipulate the mood, per se," he wrote. "It only prevents (ideally) an abnormal swing into a grossly depressive or manic state . . . but patients are free to feel any mood within the normal range at any time—just like you . . . [but] it's not foolproof, as my latest escapade illustrates. I was ON lithium (a big dose, too) during the Cherub program . . . and even so, I still had a nasty manic episode and a terrible psychotic break. So, it doesn't always work. But mainly, and theoretically, it does, so you take your lithium and try to stay out of really stressful situations, and basically cross your fingers."

Bob never reported to Miami for that internship at the *Herald*. He got out of the hospital and relapsed not long after, requiring his second hospitalization in 1986—the year that was supposed to have been the start of his brilliant career. After the second hospital stay, he decided to seek a slightly less competitive position. While he felt better again and his medication was working, he had the first of many conversations with himself about balancing wellness and career expectations.

"I think I felt I had to settle, just like I had to settle for living at home instead of a dorm," he said. "I needed something with less pressure. I wasn't sure I still had the confidence to go to a really big newspaper, try to compete for stories, and follow through on the dreams that I had.

"As a young adult, I heard the quote, 'What really matters in life is what you do with plan B.' It pretty much became my life's de facto motto."

In 1987, he took a job as a business reporter at the *News-Dispatch* in Michigan City, Indiana, close enough to Chicago that if he relapsed, his mother could help him. He did well, built up his confidence, and continued to correspond with Jon, letting him know that he felt ready to return to the faster lane. Jon was now a reporter at *The New Orleans Times-Picayune*, and his paper just happened to be on a hiring spree as Bob had finished his first year in Indiana. He recommended Bob to his editor in New Orleans.

I asked Jon, did you have any trepidation about vouching for Bob, after several major hospitalizations for manic depression?

"No, I knew he was a good guy, and I knew how talented he was," he said. "And I didn't feel that his health should be a blemish on his career, or that it should hold him back. He certainly did a great job as a reporter for four years at *The Daily Northwestern.* Why wouldn't he continue to be a great reporter?"

He did recall thinking to himself, "What am I going to say if the editor asks why he was out of work for nearly a year? And I just made up my mind that I would stick to Bob's story, that he was sick. Which was true, and all he needed to know."

Bob was hired by *The Times-Picayune* as a reporter in its East Jefferson Parish bureau in the summer of 1988, covering aviation, water pollution in Lake Ponchartrain, and the police beat. He did good work and was well regarded at the paper, but because he and Jon lived in different parts of town and worked for different bureaus, they didn't see each other all that often. Also, Jon had been there a while before Bob came, was much more social, and was in a band.

"The bottom line," Jon told me, "is that I was not a great friend to him in those first years, and I certainly didn't really think about how hard it might have been to come back after a year of struggling with his mental health and establish himself in a new city. Maybe I thought I was cool and, you know, he didn't fit—he's a big, sweet nerdy guy. I don't want to sound mean; I'm trying to be honest about myself and my own failures as a friend."

One day Jon got home from work and found a letter from Bob. He was sharing his concern that their friendship really wasn't developing, and he was disappointed. Jon, feeling guilty, went over to his apartment and they talked for several hours.

"I never had anybody confront me like that, about something like friendship," Jon told me, "and I give Bob a lot of credit. It would have been easier to just write me off as a jerk." Their friendship did improve.

It was only after that improvement that Bob told Jon he was gay.

In reality, while Bob was seeing a therapist for his manic depression, many of their sessions were about his coming out. He was twenty-five, and it was 1988, a challenging time in the gay community because AIDS was now well-known, but medical science was still six or seven years away from the first effective treatment, the protease inhibitor medications.

New Orleans was a great place to come out. "There were a lot of gay people there," Bob recalled, "and my therapist would give me homework assignments, to join organizations and meet people. I became an AIDS counselor on a hotline."

Bob changed jobs in New Orleans after several years, covering the environment and aviation for the biweekly newspaper *New Orleans CityBusiness*. And Jon moved from New Orleans to *The Dallas Morning News,* where Bob would call him on the toll-free reporters' line.

But then Bob started getting manic again. In 1991, he ended up in a hospital in New Orleans and his mother had to move down there to help him. She stayed in his apartment and visited him every day. He was psychotic for a while, and Jon, for the first time, heard on the phone what his friend was like when he was really, *really* ill.

"He would tell me he was talking to god, who told him the world was going to end," Jon recalled. "Sometimes he told me that he *was* god, but more often it was that he had spoken to god about the future, and that nuclear war was going to destroy the planet. I started writing this stuff down during these calls, because I had never heard anything like it before."

Jon remembered some of Bob's rants as being "brilliant. When he was manic, some of the stuff that came out of his mouth was profound and beautiful. Even poetic at times. And funny. He would say, 'God has a great sense of humor, although I know it's egotistical for me to say that.'"

For a while, Jon tried to talk his friend out of being psychotic. "I tried to argue with him," he said. "I remember this vividly. I would say 'Bob, you know, this is just the manic illness talking, you know that, right?' And he would explain to me why that wasn't the case. I would never get anywhere in these arguments. He was always able to outsmart me or to explain why my logic did not hold." Jon flew back to New Orleans at least once to visit Bob in the hospital.

Eventually, Bob and his mother returned to Chicago, where he was hospitalized at the Illinois State Psychiatric Institute. After recovering, he worked as a volunteer phone counselor for the LGBTQ+ Horizons HELPLINE. He also joined, and later ran, the local LGBTQ+ chapter of the national Depression and Bipolar Support Alliance (DBSA), which was one of the few exclusively gay chapters of that organization anywhere in the nation. He and his mother also became active in the Chicago chapter of Parents, Families, and Friends of Lesbians and Gays (PFLAG).

And he started going out more often, mostly to bars with karaoke, for which he developed a passion. He became a regular in Chicago karaoke—one of his favorite songs to perform was Don McLean's "American Pie," which he said the DJs really appreciated because "it's the longest song in the book, so they would call on me because they knew they could go outside and smoke."

He eventually felt well enough to return to full-time work in Chicago, writing and editing at a series of trade and business publications. First, he ran a high-priced newsletter *POS News* for the rising debit card industry for three years. Then, in the mid-1990s, he took a job writing about employee benefits for *Business Insurance* magazine. He was covering a subject close to his heart and personal insurance challenges: providing "reasonable accommodations" for disabled workers in order to retain trained employees and avoid clashing with the Americans with Disabilities Act. (This was an early version of the battle for mental health and addiction parity in insurance and employment that many of us have been fighting for over the past two decades.)

During this time, Jon Eig returned to Chicago to freelance, eventually getting a job at *Chicago* magazine. He also got married, to a fellow Northwestern grad, and began a family. Bob and his mother became members of their extended family, always invited to join them for Jewish and secular holiday meals. "His mom, Beverly, was really special," Jon remembered. "A saint who would have done anything for Bob and was just constantly there for him, advocating for him and trying to protect him through rough patches. She also made great mandel bread and stuffed cabbage." (Bob also had an older brother, Mitch, but he lived nearly three hours away at University of Illinois–Champaign where he taught broadcast journalism.)

During his four years at *Business Insurance,* Bob did something he had never done before: he told his boss he had bipolar disorder and, in an attempt to not blow up his entire life when he got symptomatic, he took medical leaves when needed. The first one came when the psychiatrist who had been overseeing his medications for the past few years, Carl Wahlstrom, began a conversation with him about the long-term side effects of lithium. He raised the possibility that Bob might need to switch to one of the antiseizure medicines that had recently been studied and used as mood stabilizers—valproate (Depakote) or carbamazepine (Tegretol), which didn't have the same toxicity to the kidneys.

Bob had already tried these medicines as part of a cocktail added to his lithium when needed, but never *instead of* the medication that had saved his life, the one he had relied on for over fifteen years. It was a nerve-racking decision to have to make, but a nephrologist they consulted said he was starting to show early signs of kidney damage. And he was experiencing epic thirst and peeing—a telltale sign of diabetes insipidus, a condition not as dangerous as regular diabetes, but challenging. So he and his doctor began the process of slowly lowering his lithium and increasing his valproate over several months.

He took what was supposed to be his last dose of lithium on July 17, 1997. Six days later, he was so manic that his mother and friends insisted he go to the emergency room at Rush Hospital. He was paranoid and delusional, convinced, among other things, that all the people in his life were "imposters"—starting with his mother who wasn't really his mother. He was discharged from the hospital, back on lithium, after two weeks. And, since he had taken a medical leave, he was soon able to return to his job.

But the issue of whether he would have to stop taking lithium hung over his care—especially since it seemed likely that without lithium, he might need to add an antipsychotic to his cocktail, and he had bad memories of his very first hospitalization and the way those meds had made him feel like a zombie. There were newer atypical antipsychotics with more focused action and less general zombification, but they had other side effects and Bob just didn't like the idea of taking them regularly. (He was not alone in this: newer atypical antipsychotics were being tried for several different diagnoses during this time, but some people just didn't want to take them.)

A year later, when Bob started getting manic again in July, Wahlstrom tried to get him to add the antipsychotic olanzapine (Zyprexa) to his cocktail. Bob refused to take it—and ended up changing doctors. He also ended up briefly hospitalized again, and not long after, he had to be weaned off lithium for good, with a higher dose of valproate and other meds to compensate.

The new cocktail worked, but never quite as well as lithium had. And his instability was increasingly challenging to his mother, who was aging and experiencing health problems of her own, having been diagnosed with thyroid cancer. So, increasingly, Jon would get calls from her asking for help. "She'd say, 'I don't know where Bob is,' or 'The police are here and they're arresting Bob,'" he recalled.

Bob remained at *Business Insurance* for four years, and after several medical leaves, he finally lost his job there. His mom's condition was getting worse, so he moved into her apartment to help her and eventually gave up his own place.

He also, for the first time, admitted to himself that he probably couldn't handle full-time employment because of his bipolar disorder. He applied for, and received, SSDI benefits.

Then his mother's illness progressed. She required a tracheotomy to allow her to keep breathing, but it sometimes got blocked in the middle of the night. Because she couldn't raise her voice anymore, she kept a bell next to her bed, which Bob knew meant he needed to jump out of bed and take her to the hospital. It would have been challenging even if he hadn't been struggling with depression.

Bob's mom died of cancer in 2001. After that, Jon got more needy phone calls from Bob. "He would call sometimes and say he ran up a big tab at a restaurant or in a cab and he couldn't pay," he recalled.

But the illness was predictably cyclical and a year later, Bob's health had improved to the point where he started looking for full-time jobs again. He got one writing for the glossy magazine of the American Medical Association (which is based in Chicago) and was able to go off disability. This ushered in a period of health stability for a few years, and also more travel than he was accustomed to, as he flew to different cities to cover AMA meetings.

He found the work interesting, especially learning about physicians' responses to the rise of managed care. He was making decent money. He also had inherited some money after he and his brother had sold their late mother's condo. And, during a previous manic episode, he had, perhaps unwisely, cashed in his 401(k) retirement account. Even with the substantial tax penalties, he had some money in the bank.

He used this period of wellness and the travel benefits of the job to do some personal traveling as well, including an extended trip to Canada.

After nearly three years at the AMA, Bob started getting manic again. He disappeared from the office for a few days and flew to Washington, where he checked into a hotel and decided he should do research at the Library of Congress for a book about Abraham Lincoln's depression. He returned home and became more obsessed with saving America and the world from nuclear destruction—a concern he had harbored since watching *Dr. Strangelove* and *Fail Safe* as a kid, but which was pushed to higher levels by his illness. He returned to Washington and rented an expensive condo, which he couldn't really afford, located between the National Cathedral and the Russian embassy. He was burning through his savings.

One day he was walking near the White House and saw a TV in a local café. "I inexplicably thought that a news channel was reporting the apparent explosion of a nuclear bomb in Russia, near Moscow," he recalled. "I was convinced that I knew the truth: that the explosion had actually been caused by an accident at a nuclear power station. I feared the event could be interpreted by either Russian officials or President George W. Bush as a deliberate hostile act and that the mistake might spur a war. I hurried to the White House and asked to speak with the 'Secret Service agent in charge.' I told a bewildered agent that I needed to be let into the White House gates because I was required to consult with Bush before the crisis turned into worldwide hostilities. They asked me for my background and I gave them my business card from the AMA, so they knew I was actually a journalist. But eventually, they just looked at me and said 'no.'"

Instead of just turning him away, Bob recalls the White House guards "put me in a nice Cadillac and they drove me to a psych hospital." Actually, they took him to one of the nation's most famous psychiatric hospitals, St. Elizabeths, which originally opened in the 1850s in response to the pioneering mental health advocacy of reformer Dorothea Dix (and was, by the time Bob got there, run down enough that it was being investigated by the Justice Department for patient rights violations). He was treated there for two weeks—during which time Secret Service agents in Illinois were sent to interview his brother and his friend Jon Eig, eventually determining he posed no threat.

Bob's brother told him the AMA magazine had reached out looking for him. "They're going to declare your job abandoned," he said.

Bob responded quickly to treatment, and then the social work staff helped him arrange a plane ticket back to Chicago. He went home and soon realized that he had spent almost all of his savings, and it was unlikely he could ever work full-time again.

He was forty-two years old and alone, with no way to support himself.

SINCE THAT TIME, Bob has been on full Social Security Disability Insurance and Medicare, Medicaid, or both. He has had many more hospitalizations for breakthrough symptoms but, as is true for many mental health patients, his stays are much shorter than such stays once were—a few days, a week or two at most, and he often feels he is being discharged too soon (and then requires readmission). Bipolar disorder involves any number of revolving doors, but he is annoyed and bewildered by how often they revolve under more managed care, with insurance companies—and in his case Medicare and Medicaid—limiting stays.

He has been fortunate that social workers have helped him find supportive residential care. For a year and a half, he lived in a private psychiatric nursing home, Greenwood Care, which was a short walk to his old Northwestern campus. When he did well there, a Chicago Housing Authority program called "Moving On" arranged for him to live in his own apartment on his SSDI benefits for nearly two years (including the first year of COVID). But money has been extremely tight. He benefited from the government giving an extra bonus during COVID to those supported by the Supplemental Nutrition Assistance Program, so his SNAP card paid for more groceries. But when his SSDI checks didn't arrive on time, he relied on community food pantries and church kitchens. Every once in a while, he tried panhandling, with little success; trying to explain that his SSDI check was late was more information than people wanted.

He did recall once getting the attention of a kind gentleman outside a grocery store who said, "I understand what you're going through," motioned him into the store, and said he could get anything he wanted for dinner. "I came away from the encounter," he said, "with a box of spaghetti, a jar of tomato sauce—and a heightened appreciation of my fellow neighbors' sense of humanity."

During these years, Bob continued to do freelance writing—some on mental health, some on nuclear disarmament issues for the Nuclear Age Peace Foundation. And he has devoted himself to volunteer work.

"I've learned over and over again that even if people with brain diseases cannot work full-time, paying jobs because of the stress, or whatever reason, they can make deeply meaningful contributions to society in other ways," he told me. "People with disabilities very often thrive on volunteer work because of the added flexibility, the reduced pressure, and the friendly, welcoming atmosphere. Volunteering can enhance the self-respect and sense of self-worth of a person with a psychiatric illness, because it proves to them that they still are needed in the world. It becomes their 'plan B.'"

Bob has tutored or taught new immigrants at Korean, Latino, Vietnamese, and South Asian community centers, educating them in the basics of English and U.S. civics to prepare them for their citizenship tests. In one of his volunteer jobs, he told me, "I accompanied two Vietnamese American teenage boys to their first baseball game ever at Chicago's Wrigley Field, and helped them order their first hot dogs." He has worked with developmentally disabled adults, teaching them the fundamentals of reading, writing, and math. For nearly a decade, he was a trained crisis line volunteer at the National Runaway Safeline, a twenty-four-hour service that offers emergency assistance to teenagers in crisis, as well as their worried parents, helping runaways get back to their families. He taught writing skills to college-bound high school seniors for the Posse Foundation.

He has also doubled down on his work in support groups for people with bipolar disorder. "Nobody—not doctors, not therapists—is in a better position to offer understanding and empathy than patients themselves," he told me. "Frequently, no one else has more valuable knowledge on symptoms, treatment, and dealing with the effects of the illness on careers, relationships, family, friends, and self-image.

Though not everyone likes peer-to-peer support, when it's successful the results can be remarkably positive."

And it is never too late to learn, or try, something new with treatment. One of the endless debates within mental health care is whether patients should be relying, primarily, on one drug that works for them, referred to as "monotherapy," or mix different medications, referred to as "polypharmacy" or a "cocktail." Bipolar patients who respond well to lithium, and don't have too many side effects, are among the most likely to choose monotherapy. But, for someone like Bob, who has relapsed so many times, the idea of adding a second or third medication—especially when there are breakthrough depression or mania symptoms—is the more modern approach, especially with newer antidepressants, antipsychotics, and secondary mood stabilizers.

Bob was forced to try something new after a manic episode neither he nor Jon Eig will ever forget. One day, Jon didn't answer the intercom phone at the front door of his condo building. Bob had been calling him so much that he just needed a break; it was also the height of COVID. Bob proceeded to call the police on his cell phone, reporting that Jon had told him he was being held at knifepoint. When the police entered his building and came banging on his apartment door, Jon had to explain that he was fine but that his bipolar friend downstairs needed help.

After this, his doctor tried adding some meds. So Bob now takes the antipsychotic aripiprazole (Abilify), to keep him from getting manic, and duloxetine (Cymbalta) to prevent depression.

In the aftermath of that mania, Bob moved back into Greenwood Care, where he spent the rest of the pandemic. In June 2022, he went to his kidney doctor—he had been monitoring his kidney issues for years after taking lithium—and a series of tests revealed problems. He also developed symptoms of colon cancer, even though he had never had an irregular colonoscopy before. He was diagnosed with stage 2 colon cancer, which was treated successfully with surgery. In the aftermath, however, his kidneys reached the point where he needed dialysis, which takes three and a half hours per session, three times a week. So he moved to a different facility, Elevate Care North Branch in the Chicago suburb of Niles—which has its own onsite dialysis center. He has lived there since.

He gets help from Jon, a handful of other devoted friends, and his brother Mitch, who bring him what he needs. "God, I can't even think of how many times I've made that run to Target," Jon said. "I get whatever's cheapest in his size: extra-large sweat pants, boxers, tube socks. And lots of T-shirts.

"I try to find the most ridiculous T-shirts just because I know it will make him laugh. If I buy him, like, a Barbie T-shirt, he'll get a kick out of that. He's a big *Star Trek* fan, so if I can find something *Star Trek,* I'll get that. Except, well, *Star Trek* sometimes factors into his manic episodes—you know, space, time. So, if he's manic, no *Star Trek*. Sports teams are safer because he doesn't really care much about sports."

As Bob looks back on sixty years, forty of them with bipolar disorder, he doesn't think so much about romantic relationships. "I have dated and had some short-term relationships," he said, "but I think I never found a long-term partner mostly because of the distraction and disruption bipolar illness brought to my life. It seemed I was devoting so much time just to staying well, avoiding the hospital, and holding on to my jobs that gaining a husband never became a front-burner priority."

But he remembers speaking at his high school graduation about his feeling that friendship was really his first concern. He said, "I hope we all have friends—not crowds of friends, just one or two loyal friends who will stay with us through it all, and that we are willing to be close to."

His friendship with Jon turned out to be one of those. And as much as he has supported Bob, the friendship has also taught Jon a lot he couldn't have learned any other way.

"It's one of the deepest relationships of my life," Jon said. "I'm incredibly thankful for him. He's a member of our family, very loving to me and my wife and our kids. But I've also seen him being put in a paddy wagon. I've been with him in emergency rooms where he had to be restrained."

He paused for a second. "I think the biggest thing I learned was how many people are struggling like this and you don't know about it. Once when I visited him in his room at Illinois Masonic Hospital in Chicago, I happened to look across the hall. And I saw a school mom I knew, just sitting in a gown in a chair watching TV. My kids were friendly with her kids. I had seen her at school. I didn't say anything to her—she was obviously going through a difficult time. But when I was leaving the floor, her husband and I just happened to get into the elevator at the same time. I wasn't sure what to say at first. But then I just told him, 'My friend is across the hall from your wife. If you ever need to talk, I'm happy to. This must be tough for you and the kids.'"

He didn't say much to Jon that day. "But he did later talk to me a couple of times just on the playground, when we were watching our kids," he recalled. "I would ask how his wife was doing, and we'd talk about what they had gone through. And I was thinking about what it would be like to learn about this for the first time just a few years into your marriage. And I guess it just made me appreciate—as I had gradually discovered with Bob—just how *normal* it is."

Chapter Nine

Naia

Naia Butler-Craig is a long way from home and hopes one day to be an incredibly long way from home—in outer space. But only if her mental health allows.

An engaging, emotional, and funny twenty-six-year-old from Orlando, Florida, Naia is an aerospace engineer in the PhD program at Georgia Tech studying spacecraft electric propulsion. She has been a NASA Space Fellow at the Jet Propulsion Laboratory in California, made the *Forbes* "30 Under 30" list in science at the age of twenty-three, and is a star in the world of women in STEM (science, technology, engineering, and mathematics). Online, she is known as @astronaia and is appreciated worldwide for her bold social media posts, as well as her leadership in the "Black in Astro" community.

But the more well-known Naia becomes in science—and the more she's honest to her online communities, and herself, about her health challenges—the more she feels that her dreams could be at risk. She has always been clear about her goal of being an astronaut. But since the very first time she sought help from a psychologist during her freshman year in college, she has been quietly cautioned that getting mental health treatment would undermine her chances of that level of professional achievement.

The student health psychologist at her college thought maybe Naia should consider trying medication, along with talk therapy, for her symptoms of anxiety, depression, panic, fear of failing, and some self-harm, cutting on her left wrist. At this suggestion, Naia wondered aloud if having a mental health medication on her medical record could hurt her chances of one day going into space. And the psychologist said that actually she had a sibling who worked at NASA, and maybe they should just ask.

So, right there during the session, she sent a text. Both Naia and the therapist assumed they would hear back that taking medication would be fine. There had been increasing news coverage about how attitudes about mental illness were finally changing, and both military and civilian pilots with mental health conditions could now train and fly as long as they got evidence-based medical care. Seeking treatment was, supposedly, no longer going to be perceived as a sign of weakness but of commitment to readiness.

They were both unpleasantly surprised when the therapist's sibling texted right back to their question about psychiatric medications with just two words:

"Avoid them."

"That's all he said," she told me. "The implication was 'Nobody is going to tell you this outright.'"

Ever since, Naia has been nervous about treatment and often scared to tell the truth about her symptoms. "I have a very bad habit of lying to my mental health providers," she said, with a grin. "Like, I would never tell them certain things for fear of having a 'psych stain' on my record."

Wait, I asked, did you say "psych stain"? Is that a thing?

"Well," she said, "that's what I call it. Look, my goal is to be an astronaut, and I know they are very strict about that. I'm hoping they release the restraints I've had to grapple with. I have lived in fear of them denying me my dream."

For years, she denied herself some of the most basic recommended care and kept most of her mental health on the down-low. Until that day in February 2023 when she saw online that one of her social media science heroes—who held a position similar to hers in the world of Black chemistry—had taken her own life at the age of twenty-eight.

"I came to the realization," Naia said, "that I can't be an astronaut if I'm dead."

NAIA BUTLER-CRAIG GREW UP in the Richmond Heights section of Orlando, the precociously bright only child of a couple who worked in hospitality—her dad as a cook for catering and food trucks, her mom in the wine business—and who split up when Naia was three. Her mom transitioned into working for their local church, St. Mark AME, which was a center of their lives.

Her parents had joint custody, and for years Naia hoped there was something she could do to bring them back together. This hope fueled her drive to do well in school, which had its advantages—high grades and achievement—but came at the cost of endless pressure and self-criticism. Her parents never had to pressure her to do well academically; she was already pressuring herself so much. She was always trying to ensure that her parents, especially her father, were proud of her. She had "frequent meltdowns" over her desire to be a good daughter.

I told her I knew a little bit about that, from my own relationship with my dad. The self-criticism felt like the only way to control my environment. I remember cheating on tests I was already going to do well on because I needed to score 100 to feel okay about myself.

She nodded, knowingly.

Naia recalled being twelve, when her father and a friend of his took her on a car trip to New York; along the way they were pulled over in South Carolina because the friend was driving erratically. When the police questioned the two men, they smelled marijuana, and somehow they determined Naia was in danger. Even though her father, who wasn't driving, was released just hours later, Naia had already been turned over to authorities and put into a temporary foster home. To make the situation even weirder and scarier, the temporary foster mother really liked her and tried to talk her into staying.

It was more than a week before Naia was able to return home, and the experience was traumatic. Growing up, she had spent time around neighborhoods with their share of poverty, violence, and substance use disasters, but that was all part of her normal. A forced foster placement at the age of twelve was not normal, and she never forgot it.

Not long after, she realized it was time to stop hoping her parents would get back together. "I was old enough to give up on that dream," she said.

The next year, she experienced another traumatic event. "Another friend of my dad—who, like most of his friends, were like my uncles—was murdered in his home," she recalled. "He was actually holding his child when he got shot. It was a very crazy situation, and his daughter was my best friend, and so that night my dad went to their house to pick up the family's stuff for them, and I went with him. And it was a fresh crime scene. He told me not to come in, to stay in the car, but I wanted to be supportive of my dad, so I went in with him. He was, like, 'You make that decision, you can't turn back, and you may see something crazy.' I saw the fresh blood on the floor but, truthfully, I remember this being more about helping and supporting my dad. He's strong for everyone else and I wanted to be strong for him."

As she got older, Naia continued doing very well in school. But she told me, "Privately, I just felt like I did everything wrong. I did not like myself." When she was alone, she would sometimes lose control of her emotions, with explosive crying and meltdowns. She decided to start staying mostly at her mother's house, visiting her dad on weekends.

The first time anyone else saw her lose control like this was during Christmas when she was fifteen. She and her mother had driven down to the church and left all of Naia's Christmas gifts in a bag in the back seat of the car.

"We were at the church pretty late, and someone broke into our car," she recalled. "My mom heard smashing glass, looked out the church window, and saw somebody running off with the stuff she bought me for Christmas. And I was *begging* her not to go, it was dangerous. But she's very stubborn and she wouldn't listen to me. She immediately went chasing after them, yelling, 'You will not ruin my child's Christmas!' So she's down the street, and they finally drop the gifts. But in the meantime, I'm back at the church hyperventilating and when she comes back, she finds me having an anxiety attack."

When Naia was sixteen, she got her first bad grade ever—a D on a chemistry test, which to her meant she "failed"—and she came home and started what she referred to as "snowballing," during which her emotions escalated until she was totally out of control. At the peak of it, she picked up a razor blade and cut her left wrist.

"I don't remember that I was trying to kill myself," she recalled.

"It was just really a way to stop the meltdown from getting any worse." In fact, she actually remembered thinking, just before lowering the blade to her skin, that she had seen an episode of the cartoon *Family Guy* where a character made a joke about how to self-harm, saying "sideways for attention, long way for results." And while she didn't feel that she was doing this for attention at all—she was just really upset with herself—she did cut herself "sideways," horizontally, and not "for results." She just bled a lot until she calmed down and bandaged herself.

Nobody else knew about the cutting until almost a year later when, after having an argument with her mom, she went to her room, took a handful of pills, and cut her wrist. "She found me on the floor," Naia recalled, "razor blade in hand, blood on wrist, pills surrounding me. I don't know what I was thinking but I just kinda had a meltdown because she was upset with me and I wasn't used to her being upset with me. This was still early in my . . . well, I hate to call it a 'journey' of doing that, of cutting myself."

I asked her why she thought she was cutting herself.

"I remember, and this is something that stuck with me, I felt like I *deserved* it," she said. "My mom thought I got the idea from a friend and that I did it because I was influenced. But I just remember wanting to punish myself because I struggled with a lot of self-hatred. I mean, I still struggle with this today."

At the time, it didn't occur to Naia or to her mother that she needed help. "I try not to worry my mom a lot of the time," she said. "Like, we do a lot of trying to spare each other."

Naia had no mental health treatment until she got to college, where she was on scholarship at Embry-Riddle Aeronautical University in Daytona Beach, about an hour from her home. She thought the therapy she received from a student health psychologist was valuable. But after the therapist texted her sibling, who suggested a psychiatric medication prescription could hurt her chances of being an astronaut, Naia started thinking about other things she might not want on her record—such as her periodic feelings of anxiety, panic, and depression, or her suicidal ideation. So, she decided it was okay to sometimes bend the truth when talking to mental health professionals, and even occasionally okay to flat out lie.

This happens more often than people realize and can seem relatively benign—until it isn't. That's especially true when a patient believes it's safe not to share feelings having to do with self-harm and suicidality. The very act of sharing these symptoms—and they are symptoms, no matter how much they can feel like existential truths—can often save lives.

Even after the discouraging message from her sibling at NASA, Naia's psychologist did convince her to at least meet with a primary care physician who could evaluate her and maybe write her a prescription for an antidepressant. He asked about her history and Naia admitted to cutting because he could see the scars on her wrist. She told him she had been doing it since high school.

"Didn't your parents know?" he asked.

She told him they had found out.

"And they didn't take you to counseling?"

She recalled feeling insulted by the way he asked. "He, like, scoffed, and I tried to explain, 'No, they didn't know to do that.' And I didn't like that he didn't understand the nuance of the Black community when it came to mental health. So that pissed me off."

Did you feel he was criticizing you or your parents?

"Well," she said, "I'm very protective of my parents."

I told her it sounded like she was sometimes more protective of them than she was of herself.

"That's true," she laughed. "Definitely true. And still true."

The doctor wrote her a prescription for fluoxetine (Prozac, which is, actually, one of a handful of psychiatric medications that pilots and training pilots, civilian and military, are now technically allowed to use). But she never filled it. She never went back to him and never told the psychologist she hadn't filled it.

SOCIAL MEDIA HAD not played a huge part in Naia's life during high school. But when she got to college in 2015, she saw how much the STEM world communicated through what was then called Twitter, along with Instagram. So she started posting and building an online presence. As @astronaia, she networked with scientists all over the world who watched her grow into a bold combination of enthusiastic jet propulsion nerd, diversity advocate, fashion diva, and emotional confessor. Since she had such a large following, it was surprising—even to Naia—how much of her life and struggles she was able to keep secret.

She continued to have periodic meltdowns, anxiety attacks, episodes of cutting, and powerful suicidal ideation all through this time in the jet propulsion and social media spotlight. For many years she made some passing references to what was going on with her, rarely using words that would make it clear she wasn't just having "issues" or "problems" but serious mental health symptoms, which she was only partially treating for fear of losing her chance to be in space.

During her senior year in college, she finally started being more honest with her therapist about her symptoms, accepted a diagnosis of panic disorder, and decided to apply to the school's disability office for a mental health "accommodation." This allowed her a little extra time taking tests and a little more leeway with other assignments if she was not feeling well.

"I was definitely a little bit embarrassed by it," she recalled, "especially because I don't have, like, an outwardly visible disability. I didn't want people questioning me and thinking I was trying to take an easy way out. I was just trying to survive." She was given another prescription for Prozac but was still afraid that filling it would show up on her record, so she didn't. By this time, she already had her first relationship with NASA: she started as a Pathway Systems Engineer intern with the NASA Glenn Research Center in Ohio, working on projects remotely. But she wanted to make sure that when she applied to be in space for NASA there wouldn't be any problems.

The semester went well enough, as did her applications to graduate school for PhD programs in jet propulsion. On December 30, 2018, as she headed into her final college semester, she posted the news that she had been accepted into the MS/PhD program at Georgia Institute of Technology in Atlanta with a full-ride scholarship, along with other good news from the past year: "Published twice . . . NSBE Region of the year . . . Presented at two AIAA conferences . . . Started a business . . . Fired my first electric thruster . . . Launched my first spacecraft."

But then, the next day—at 1:37 A.M. on New Year's Eve—she added this response to the first post:

"I should also mention: I failed my first class, fell back into self-harm, had serious $$ issues, had major anxiety attacks, faced A LOT of self doubt. But I grew so much because of it. I had a great support system and I can't thank them enough. thankful for the good & bad." It was the first time she offered more than a hint of what she was experiencing.

Some friends were still awake at that hour and responded. Naia wrote back, "My faith has grown exponentially. God showed me just how intentional he is . . . I failed a major aerospace class—thought my life was over—and got into Georgia Tech in the same year. Proof that you should never give up!"

After graduation in the spring, she was so certain she was done cutting herself that she had the word "Beyond" tattooed on the inside of her left wrist. A month later, she posted about that: "something I've been reluctant to share but am willing to be vulnerable . . . my beyond tattoo is tattooed over where I used to self-harm. This is my declaration that I'm beyond the circumstances that cause me to do that. Never again."

It was the first of many "never agains."

NAIA SOMETIMES TOLD her psychologist when she cut herself and when she was feeling suicidal. She never thought of cutting as suicidal, because when she imagined taking her own life, that was never the way she did it. Instead, she imagined herself "overdosing on pills, or driving my car off something, or just . . . well, I know we're talking about it to *help,* but to me it's still a little vulgar to say: okay, I thought about just shooting myself."

And when she had those thoughts, she needed to take some action for self-protection. Because, as her psychologist knew, "I do own a firearm, and I'm licensed to carry."

I asked if her decision to carry a gun was driven by any specific incident at school.

"No," she said. "I was raised with my dad always taking me to the gun range. And when I was able to purchase one of my own, it was more about protection. I'm a young lady. I've been living by myself since I was seventeen. I go to all these internships and I'm in different cities. My personal safety as a young single woman was always important to me." She has always kept her pistol disassembled and locked away. And whenever she felt a return of the ideation, she would give it to a friend to hold.

The summer after she graduated, Naia went to New Mexico, where she had been selected for a prestigious internship at Los Alamos National Laboratory, the remote research facility originally developed for the Manhattan Project. She was mentored there by computational astrophysicist Nicole Lloyd-Ronning, who was amazed by her ability to quickly absorb science that was new to her. "Naia came here as an engineer with really no plasma physics training, and no code training," she said, "and within a week she was having the code up and running and getting results. She was phenomenal."

Naia was also resilient, and that proved to be necessary. Early in her summer at Los Alamos, a fellow young scientist said a "horrible racist thing to Naia," Nicole recalled. He said that Naia was more likely to get a job than he was because she was "a Black girl" and he was white.

Nicole, who is also white, was incensed when she heard this comment. "I mean, I wanted to punch him," she recalled. "All I did in the moment was say that wasn't true. It is never easier at this moment in our history, or anytime until now, for a Black woman to get a job." When he left, Naia hugged Nicole and thanked her for saying that.

WHEN SHE ARRIVED at Georgia Tech for graduate school in the fall of 2019, Naia was less apologetic about applying for a disability accommodation for her psychiatric diagnosis—which the mental health professional who saw her there changed to generalized anxiety disorder.

"Getting this disability accommodation," she said, "really made me reflect on how many Black students don't even know that those things are available to them or are too underdiagnosed to even be exposed to the idea of disability accommodations." The psychiatrist who helped her get the accommodation also wrote her a prescription for Prozac. Again, she didn't take it.

Her first year of grad school was interrupted by COVID in the spring, so she started learning remotely. She became more politically active on social media after the death of George Floyd and the Black Lives Matter protests. Some of her followers supported this, while others suggested that "Black scientists don't have the luxury of tweeting about inflammatory things." She let them know she could "walk and chew gum at the same time."

In December 2020, she was named one of *Forbes* magazine's "30 Under 30" in science. "While this award does not validate me," she posted, "I am grateful to be recognized." This led to other media opportunities, as well as more academic and public pressure.

In the spring of 2021, as people were beginning to be vaccinated and start interacting again, her anxiety, cutting, and suicidal ideation became concerning enough that she did something shocking. On April 19, 2021, she went to therapy and told the truth, the whole truth.

Later that day she posted, "Um so shout out to me. I did something I consider super brave today. I was totally honest with my mental health care provider! I've always held back in therapy due to concerns of hindering my future career (astronaut). But today I decided that my mental health matters more."

Over the next year, she continued doing well academically and professionally, but she struggled personally. She became more active on social media. She got more attention for her work in the lay and scientific media but had other challenges. Her father got cancer and, though his treatment was ultimately successful, she was extremely worried. She made a mistake filing her taxes and owed money she didn't have. Then she found out that her birth control had failed and she was pregnant. Within a week she had a miscarriage, which required an emergency room visit. She flunked her first grad school class that semester, the course in viscous fluid flow.

And then she went to Pasadena, California, where she had been accepted for a three-month internship at the NASA Jet Propulsion Laboratory—a "very big deal, and I had no idea the topics I was going to be working on there," she remembered. "It was like the steepest learning curve ever."

While in that heady environment, she also had to study for her "quals," the crucial, two-day qualifying exams for her PhD, which were done orally, just her in a room with proctors. "Our format," she noted, "is super hard and Georgia Tech is extremely notorious for its supernatural exams."

She got back to Georgia at the end of the summer, was cramming for her quals, and trying everything not to lose control. She still didn't want to take medication, remaining too afraid it could dash her astronaut dreams just as she was getting closer. With two weeks left before she had to take her exam, she had a friend take away her locked-up gun. She was feeling more and more suicidal by the hour.

"I was flirting with the idea," she told me. "I was feeling serious urges, which made it very hard to trust myself. I was afraid of my own mind, afraid of myself. And so, it was to the point where I was trying to rationalize me dying. I'm thinking, 'Maybe this is what God wants. Maybe this makes sense.' I had the thought that death looked better to me than failure, because I had married my life to my career so badly.

"The thoughts were getting that deep, and they had never gotten that deep before. This happened first when I was at home studying, and then I thought maybe being home was driving me kinda nuts. And then I went to a restaurant and I sat there and tried to study. And then I kind of panicked. My heartbeat was racing. I went out to my car and thought about it."

She texted one of her closest friends, "who I had been telling about everything." It was her friend's idea that she should go to the nearest hospital emergency room and ask for help. They texted back and forth about the pros and cons of Naia seeking treatment, after she had worked so hard—and probably suffered so much unnecessarily—just to avoid having a mental health prescription, a "psych stain," on her medical record. Her friend finally convinced her to drive to the hospital.

Naia called her mother on the way there. She thought they would take her phone if she voluntarily went in for emergency psychiatric care, and "I knew my mom would, literally, call in an airstrike if she couldn't contact me." She was worried that her mother might try to talk her out of it, but "she was very supportive." It turned out the hospital did not have a psychiatric unit, so she had to decide what to do next. The physician who had seen her in the ER during her miscarriage was actually on call and came to talk to her. Knowing her background, he wanted to make sure she realized what she was doing. In order for her to be transported to a psychiatric hospital, he would have to sign what, in the state of Georgia, was called a 1013, which meant she was an "imminent danger" to herself or others, or she was unable to care for her own health and safety.

She told him she honestly didn't know what else to do. "I was telling them the truth," she recalled, "which was not standard for me, because I knew what the consequences were for telling the truth.

And he was, like, 'Well, okay then.' And then they just left me. Some of the people seemed angry at me. But I would say the Black nurses, they were checking on me and making sure I was okay."

NAIA WAS TRANSFERRED to nearby Peachford psychiatric hospital. Her first hours there were under suicide watch, so someone was with her even when she went to the bathroom. But then she got a room. She had just turned twenty-five and felt like the oldest person on the unit. She remembered one fifteen-year-old who was "warning me about 'booty juice,' which is what they call the stuff they stick in your butt when you're acting out too much. None of that happened with me. I was more scared than anything. They ended up putting me on Lexapro and something to help me sleep."

I asked how she felt once she was in the unit and, presumably, out of immediate danger.

"I was mostly scared because my exams were the following week," she said, "and they wouldn't let anybody bring me my textbooks so I could study, at least, while I was there. And they wouldn't let me have my iPad. So I was, literally, using colored pencils and printer paper to draw out what I could from memory. That was the only thing that made me feel like I had made a mistake. I was really scared about that. Otherwise, I knew I had done the right thing for my health."

When she had been at Peachford for a week, she realized she might not get out in time to take her exams. She had already deferred them once, and if she didn't take them, she could flunk out and lose her scholarship. She had talked to one of her Georgia Tech advisers in the past about some of her mental health challenges, but she had never led him to believe it was bad enough that she might call him from a psychiatric hospital. So she was reluctant to reach out. Finally on Sunday, the day before her exams were to start, she was able to call him.

She was surprised when he was sympathetic—because she had been so unrelenting with herself. "He was, like, 'Why are you even calling me?'" she recalled. "'You need to be focused on your health.'" Her tests were deferred until the first of the year, and she finished her nine-day stay in the hospital.

When she got home and reconnected with her regular therapist and psychiatrist, they decided to make a few changes in her medications. Her psychiatrist decided she needed a stronger medication than just the antidepressant she had been taking since the hospitalization and gave her a prescription for Prozac as well as the antipsychotic medicine quetiapine (Seroquel).

This helped some, but she also noticed she was developing a very unsettling tic, where her head would repeatedly cock slightly but sharply to the left. She recorded herself doing it on her phone to show to the doctor, who decided it was a stress reaction.

But by the holidays, she was feeling more anxious and suicidal again.

"So I have not shared this anywhere," she told me, "but that December I tried to overdose on my antipsychotic medicine. I took all the pills, and then I tried to take all my antidepressants, too. Everything appeared in slow motion all the sudden, and I got super, like, slurring all my words. But I was able to just spit most of it up."

So I asked, who did you finally tell about this?

"No one," she said. "You. Just now."

You never told your mental health professional?

"No, because I had the test coming up again in January," she admitted, "and I was afraid if I told her, she would make me go back to the hospital, and then I would fail."

Nobody knew a thing about this attempt—unless they were able to read between the lines of her social media posts. On the day after Christmas, at 9:07 A.M., she posted:

"Random but having to choose between life-saving mental health resources / quality of life and your career, sucks."

Of course, now she was out of pills. What, I wondered, did you tell your doctor happened to your pills so you could get more?

"I told her I dropped them," she said, "and I got them refilled."

She didn't feel quite normal yet after the overdose, so she asked her mom to come stay with her and help her until after the quals.

Two weeks later, Naia took her qualifying exams. The quals are done in a classroom—all questions are posed orally by a group of three professors. The first day she felt she was barely holding it together, but she did make it through. She returned the second day feeling much worse—teary and panicky before even coming into the room. About a third of the way through the oral exam, she got up, crying, said she had to leave, and tried to walk out. But one of her professors stopped her and convinced her to stay. She was able to calm down and finish the rest of the test.

She later found out that she had failed the test on the first day but, miraculously, passed the second day. So, she was allowed to continue in the program, and would get one more chance to pass.

SEVERAL WEEKS LATER, Naia recorded a video of herself on her iPhone talking very openly about suicide. She decided not to post it. While her mental health was still perilous, she felt she had already jeopardized her future as an astronaut enough by being hospitalized and taking medication. She had several STEM friends who had flown in space with private companies, such as SpaceX and Blue Origin. She wondered if private space travel could be a plan B.

But she knew that wasn't what she wanted. NASA and its values of scientific progress and discovery were her ultimate dream. "When I go into space," she said, "I want to actually support a mission."

She wasn't sure what to do with the very honest video. So she just let it sit in her iPhone for a while.

At the beginning of February 2023, Black in Astro, the group of Black astronomy academics of which Naia was a board member, was honored by the Royal Astronomical Society for its "dedication to fostering joy and authenticity for all Black people interested in STEM [which] sets it apart from most outreach initiatives." Naia was thrilled.

But three weeks later, she was devastated to learn that Samantha "Sammy" Mensah, the doctoral candidate in chemistry at UCLA who was one of Naia's role models for Black STEM leadership, had taken her own life. As suicide prevention messages for young scientists began deluging social media, Naia went back to the video she had made about her hospitalization. She started editing it down on her iPhone.

In the two-minute video she cut, she is sitting in her bedroom, weepy in a red tank top, explaining, "I decided to use all the resources that were available to me . . . to stay here. Because, bottom line, if I am not alive I cannot be an astronaut. If I am not here, I cannot reach my dreams."

Her emotional declaration was reinforced in bold, capital letters below her face.

"I'm still living with those decisions and navigating those decisions," she continued, tearing up, "because it may be the case that I did forfeit my dream. But it'll be okay, because I surrendered my plans to who I recognize as my God, and I trust my god. So whatever he, or she, or they might have in store for me is much greater than I ever could have imagined . . .

"This is my journey. It may not look like how I thought it was gonna look . . . and I may not feel as smart as Sally, Sue, Mary and Joe, but this is mine, it is all mine. It is my journey and I'm going to walk through it as I need to. And if I get to that finish line, who gives a hoot about how long it took me or about how I got there. As long as its moral and ethical, baby, a PhD is a PhD, a degree is a degree. C's get degrees . . . period point blank. So . . ." And then it just trailed off.

Before posting it to Twitter, she tagged it "TW"—shorthand for "trigger warning"—and "suicidal ideation." And then she wrote, in a series of connected posts, "This is me discussing how I started anti-depressants after avoiding them for years for the sake of my career . . . and how I ended up in a mental health facility which also poses a risk to my dreams since mental health is still very much stigmatized in flight careers and the aerospace industry in general. . . . This is not me encouraging or discouraging medication. It's just an example of how I decided to prioritize my quality of life over my lofty goals of being a space explorer. Doing so played a huge part in sending me into a really deep depressive episode."

She then concluded, "We r losing 2 many to suicide. & you never know what it is that created that hopelessness in a person. what I do know is many of us are trying to navigate systems that r not built for us. & we blame ourselves for not succeeding in the traditional ways that these systems encourage"

And then she posted it.

The post, and several follow-ups, got a lot of attention, over 30,000 views. "A lot of people saw it. And I think it was taken as 'Okay, you can't kick me out of NASA if I'm a mental health advocate.' As for me, I was worried that I had just handed them my disqualification on a platter."

But she had, by posting more truth, finally freed herself to actually be treated more fully and share more with her mental health professionals. She had an intriguing session with her therapist after posting it. "She told me she thought it was really admirable that I had posted it," she recalled, "but she said, 'That doesn't mean I think you should have done it.'" The psychologist especially thought Naia should have waited to post it until after discussing it in a therapy session.

By spring, Naia was posting more details of her care on social media, and even having a little fun with it—she made a video of herself in a little skit, pretending to struggle to answer the questions during her qual.

Her improved health helped her through more challenges. On May 3, 2023, her cousin, Calvin Craig, who she always thought of as an older brother, was discovered murdered in his home. He was thirty-three.

"It was a grisly thing, and in the news," she said. "And the purpose of me bringing it up is to shed light on the duality of my life. Obviously, I'm in academia, I'm doing these interesting, cool, kind of niche-special things. But I'm still a Black woman, and the things that ail the Black community I still very much feel on a personal level. And I think that makes my journey so complex. Cause I had to deal with that and then I went to his funeral. I had to *plan* his funeral actually. Went home, bought the bouquets and all that stuff, did the program. And then, you know, the next week I'm right back in the lab, trying to get research done."

While she was pleased that her stronger commitment to treatment and honesty about her illness was helping, she did notice one thing she never would have expected making things harder: the many changes in Twitter as it changed ownership and rebranded as X. There has been much written about how social media platforms can influence mental health in negative ways, by creating a forum for spreading rumors and embarrassing images, bullying, even creating contagion for self-harm and suicidality. But social media can also serve as a coping mechanism, and over the years Naia has made many friends she only knew from public tweets and private Direct Messages.

Over the years, Twitter had become a place where several of the marginalized groups she represented were able to find one another from around the world; responses of support could be expected at any hour, day or night. But after Twitter was sold and its content monitoring eliminated, many of the people she knew from all those worlds stopped posting or even closed their accounts.

As she has grown into a cross-platform "influencer," Naia now posts more on TikTok and Instagram, and includes more videos and visuals, which those sites encourage. But as she recently wrote, "I miss the twitter days of old so bad. My twitter family was everything as I was navigating the school stuff."

When we met, Naia was in the middle of rethinking whether being open about her mental health care really needed to end her dream of flying for NASA. She was feeling stronger and healthier than she had in years, and more convinced than ever that if NASA tried to keep her from being an astronaut because of her mental illness—now well treated—she was ready to raise her voice about it.

I told her I was ready to raise mine, too. In my years of working to make sure there is broad social and legal support for mental health care and reimbursement, I have talked to everyone from the chairman of the Joint Chiefs of Staff on down in the military about these issues, as well as many leaders in civil aeronautics. They have been very clear, for quite a while now, that mental health treatment was now considered a crucial cornerstone of "operational readiness."

I started telling Naia about the first time I heard this directly from a military leader—at the John F. Kennedy Special Warfare Center and School at Fort Liberty, talking to General Hugh Shelton about mental health care for Green Berets. He said that Special Ops had the best mental health care of any other branch of the service. "We don't look at mental health care as a safety net," he said. "We look at it as a force multiplier."

She was surprised to hear this. "That is *so good* to know," she said.

Of course, as I know too well, there can be a big difference between an organization's political position on mental health and how individual people are actually treated when they need it. I let her know that if she wanted to be even more public in her advocacy, I had her back.

As our series of conversations wound down, Naia let me know she was going to have to disappear for a few weeks. Her final chance to pass her last qual was coming, as was her twenty-sixth birthday. She was going to do nothing but study until the test, and then she was going to go on her first real vacation while awaiting the results that would determine her entire future.

On September 30, 2023, at 10:15 P.M., she went to Twitter and posted just five words:

"Friends. I finally passed quals." It was followed by three emojis: a weeping face, a half-smiling face with teary eyes, and then a smiling face with just a single tear. 😭 🥹 🥲

Chapter Ten

Gene, Gretchen & Tommy

I have been listening to people talk openly and powerfully about their addictions for decades: at twelve-step meetings; in long, teary phone calls; at conferences; during legislative testimony; or just privately, pulling me aside.

But none of this really prepared me for the forty-nine minutes I spent talking with Gretchen Ficek, a fifty-eight-year-old woman who raised two daughters in Colorado while working in telecommunications and holding precariously to her sobriety—but who had, for the past two years, been experiencing homelessness, living next to a dumpster behind a Walmart in Santee, California, not far from San Diego.

"I'm choosing to drink and use drugs," she told me, her voice strong and determined. "That makes no sense to me. Because the way I'm living now it's just sad. It's just . . . it's just wrong. I know I should be doing more with my life. And I just don't want to. And for me not to want to . . . well, that's what's crazy to me."

It had taken over a year to arrange to speak to Gretchen. The conversation took place on her shaky cell phone, just an hour before she had to check out after a brief stay in a hotel room. It had been arranged by her father because her boyfriend had been arrested and the weather was terrible.

Her father is a colleague of mine, semiretired tech entrepreneur Gene Barduson, who had a big career at IBM during the '60s and '70s as a top sales and management executive, then started and sold a handful of tech companies of his own, before moving into health-care technology companies and then medical philanthropy. He recently started a nonprofit hoping to revolutionize research on addiction—because he has personally experienced four generations of struggles with substance use.

Gene suffered from alcoholism all through the first decades of his professional life—and it went largely unnoticed in the after-work party culture at IBM. He got sober at the age of forty-five with the help of rehab, AA, and a very supportive wife. And then he watched some of his family succeed professionally, only to have nearly everything taken away by addiction.

One of his sons, Tommy, an internet sports executive, died in his early fifties from multiple organ failure caused by his intense and unrelenting alcohol use.

And Gretchen, the elder of his two daughters, is still, every day, deciding her own fate.

A smart, athletic young woman, Gretchen was recruited to work at Sprint in Denver right after graduating from the University of Northern Colorado. She married and, after seven years with the company, became a stay-at-home mom. She struggled with her drinking, and when her daughters were young she went to rehab. "And I stayed sober for seven and a half years, because I wanted to, because I wanted to be there for my children," she told me. "And then the marriage started to get bad, and I just didn't want it anymore. And I didn't want to stay sober."

She went back to Sprint and did her best to balance family and career while struggling with alcohol and then hydrocodone (Vicodin), which was initially prescribed for migraines, then misused. She explained that she lost her job ostensibly because she gave a friend at work one of her Vicodin when he wasn't feeling well—and someone reported it. She initially made it sound like that had been unfair but then admitted that she had not been in good health.

"I worked in corporate America for seventeen years, throughout the years my kids were growing, and, you know, held a job and did all that," she said. "I don't know, I just *lived*. And, I mean, it's weird because now I'm not living. I feel like I'm just existing. And that's a problem. I'm an alcoholic. So I used to drink. And now I *drink all the time*." In the past ten years, she has been in prison twice, and detox and rehab several times.

Her daughters, both in their twenties, won't communicate with her until she gets sober. "Mom," they say, "we can't sit and watch you die."

"We have what I guess you could call a beautiful relationship, because they still love me and accept me," she said. "But they will not have anything to do with me. I cannot see them. They won't be around me if I'm using and that's fair. Those are their boundaries."

Gretchen has incredibly mixed feelings about her father—who supported her for years after she stopped working, even as she spent much of her time drinking in an apartment he paid for. She knows he was encouraged to do this by her mother, who urged Gene to continue subsidizing Gretchen's life, even though he worried it was too enabling.

But after her mom died in early 2018, her father let her know that if she didn't get help, he wouldn't keep supporting her forever. And after several more attempts at helping her get sober, he finally, to her absolute astonishment, stopped paying for her apartment in the fall of 2019. Gretchen began staying with a boyfriend who was already experiencing homelessness himself.

"I never thought in a million years he'd ever do that," she admitted. "And he told me what was going to happen and I just didn't believe him. Because he had always taken care of me. But it's just a part of tough love. He's not gonna sit there and watch me die. I understand that. It just hurts a lot. It's just really hard to deal with. But those were my choices. So he's very . . . well, he helps me when he can." She sighed.

"You know I'm in a wheelchair now," she told me. I couldn't see her—she hadn't been able to load Zoom onto her phone—so I wouldn't have known otherwise. Six months earlier, she had been walking across a multilane highway, high on meth. She got as far as the median, and when she tried to step off of it, a food delivery car slammed into her and dragged her across three lanes of traffic.

"I broke my neck and my back and my pelvis and my legs, from the knees down," she said. "And I have to say, God wants me on this earth for some reason, and I'm figuring out what it is—because all the doctors who have done all the surgeries and all this stuff, say, 'Gretchen, you should be dead. If you're not dead, you should be paralyzed from the neck down.' So there's a reason I'm on this earth. And I just need to get out of this hole that I'm in and just do better."

I asked what had worked for her in the past, even if it only worked temporarily.

"Well, it's *desire*," she said. "Just the desire to stay clean and sober. And right now, it's easier for me to stay drunk and high. And that makes no sense to me. But that's what it is."

Suddenly she said, "I hate to cut this short, but I have to pack up and get out of here."

I didn't want to let her hang up. "Thank you so much, Gretchen. I'm an alcoholic myself, so I totally relate," I said. "It took me thirty years of drinking and drugging before I got sobriety. I had to leave my job, leave where I lived. Leave everybody I knew. All I had were meetings, three or four times a day for a year. And then it started getting easier. But I know exactly how overwhelming the feeling is. Starting down that road seems really insurmountable. But you have great insight into how desperate your situation is. And that really is important."

She said she appreciated that. "The fact that you even want to chat with me is huge," she said. "So thank you for everything and please reach out to me again, or I'll reach out to you, either way, but I'd love to continue the conversation."

The phone line went dead. I haven't heard from her since.

GENE BARDUSON CEASED to be shocked a long time ago by the amazing power of addiction. He's now in his early eighties, and I'm glad he was willing to share his story. It's often hard to appreciate just how tirelessly families struggle to protect their loved ones with substance use disorders—because people are so good at hiding it.

Gene grew up on a farm near a small town in western Minnesota, Big Bend City, where his father struggled with alcohol.

"He would stay sober for weeks, even a couple of months, to attend to the farm," he explained, "and then he would disappear for two, three, four days." He recalls that as a young boy, he would search the barn and the hay lofts for his father's bottles, and then take them to the creek and smash them against the rocks, cursing alcohol and swearing he would never drink. His father would sometimes get treatment at what they called "the crazy house," a mental health center eighty miles away, but he struggled to maintain sobriety. In the 1960s, his father went to Hazelden, the historic alcohol treatment center outside of Minneapolis that was founded after World War II on the precepts of Alcoholics Anonymous (and which is now part of the Hazelden Betty Ford Foundation). For the last four decades of his life, "he remained sober and became known as the father of AA in our community, and anybody who had any problems came to him." He died at the age of ninety-six.

Gene didn't drink or smoke through high school because it was the surest way to get thrown off a sports team, and football, basketball, and especially baseball were his life. He attended North Dakota State University. He had his first beer at a fraternity in 1958, "and I never stopped drinking after that." But he was able to balance drinking with his schoolwork. He graduated and taught high school for several years outside Minneapolis. He married a fellow teacher, Mary, and then, after they had two sons he got a scholarship to go to grad school in mathematics at the University of Northern Iowa. He was hired by IBM in 1966, first on the technical side and then on the sales side, beginning in Iowa City but later moving around the country.

"They had strict rules about drinking during work hours," he recalled, "and we were given incredible responsibility because there was no computer generation before us. We were 'IBM people'—you know, black suits, white shirts, ties. But at night, there was a lot of partying and drinking. Pretty much everybody I spent the next sixteen years with in the offices did a lot of drinking: weeknights, weekends. It was almost expected."

He miraculously survived a number of alcohol-related accidents. "I totaled three cars, met up with two bridges. Nobody said anything. The next day we went and had the car towed—no investigation, no nothing. I just got a different car," he said. His wife, whose father had been an alcoholic, was one of the few people in his life who expressed fear of what he was doing. "She was constantly wanting me to be different," he said. "I was missing kids' games, things that I regret and am ashamed about. I was just focused on the work, and drinking was sort of the oil that made me do it. Yet, it did get worse, and it became harder to do my job."

I was curious to know if there was a time when he believed he couldn't continue working at that level without drinking.

"No, no, I always thought it was something that was going to get in my way," he said. "Privately, I used to pray every day, 'Please, lift this curse from me.'"

By then, Gene and Mary had four kids—two sons and Gretchen, who had been born just a year or so apart, and then another daughter, five years later, who was almost raised as an only child. After sixteen years at IBM, he cashed out and did what many were doing—using their IBM credibility to help create a new generation of tech start-ups. He got involved with one in Salt Lake City on the cutting edge of computer-assisted design and manufacturing. The company ended up firing him in 1985—in part because he was on the wrong side of a board split, but the new CEO later told him that it was also because of his drinking. The last straw had been a flight back from a Tokyo business meeting, during which Gene got so drunk he needed to be helped off the plane, and Mary had to come and get him.

"The CEO said, 'I know you have a problem. But I will give you great references wherever you want to go,'" he recalled. "And he did give me a terrific reference and a great severance package and I had a job within, probably, a month."

One morning at breakfast, Mary pointed out in the newspaper that a new rehab hospital had opened in Salt Lake, called Highland

Ridge. "It's just for executives," she said, "and it's just down the street. Do you want to go?" And for the first time, he said, "Yes."

He checked in for a thirty-day program. But after several weeks, he got restless. He called friends in Salt Lake from the rehab and tried to arrange a party, with alcohol, for the day he got out. Instead, "the next morning," he told me, "I woke up, I looked in the mirror, and said, 'I'm never going to drink again.' And I never have."

When they told their college-age children that their dad was going to rehab, the news was met with shock. That made Gene feel even worse—his substance use and absence had become so normalized that his kids no longer even considered that family life could be any different.

Gretchen told me she remembered, "I was eighteen years old, my mom called and she said that Dad went to rehab. And I'm, like, 'Why?' I didn't think there was a problem at all. When that's the life you're living every day, you don't know anything else. And that's when all of us learned about alcoholism."

Gene didn't go to meetings every day as some people do: after leaving residential care, he went to one "after care" meeting a week with counselors from the program, and one or two AA meetings. He attended a couple meetings a week for the better part of two decades, and he still goes, although less frequently.

"I would have had more balance in my life if I had participated more actively in AA," he admitted. "But I'm pretty damn stubborn. So when I said I wasn't drinking anymore, I just *didn't*."

Some people are able to do this successfully—just stop. Yet that fact sometimes makes things even more confusing and challenging for those of us who are unable to remain sober without meetings or other regular support. And I think not having ongoing support or treatment often makes things more nerve-racking for family members worried about relapsing.

None of this was easy on his wife, Mary. "God bless her, she stayed with me through all this stuff, which isn't always the case," he said. "She was an incredible person and devoted to the kids. She was compassionate, sometimes very angry—and I don't blame her for that. But I was very lucky."

Once sober, Gene worked in Salt Lake City for another tech start-up and then cofounded a consulting firm, before he and Mary moved to Chicago in the early 1990s and he shifted his focus to health care. He took a senior VP job at a company run by former IBM colleagues to provide computer-based information processing for health-care providers. In 1995, he left to become CEO of a computerized medical transcription firm. He was, by then, ten years sober and trying to help his kids stay the same way.

GENE AND MARY'S second son, Tommy, had chosen a completely different career path than his father but later developed a similar struggle with alcohol. Tommy was very companionable, sometimes quiet but bright and witty. After graduating in 1987 from the University of Colorado Boulder with a degree in finance, he was hired into the management training program at GTE Financial, where he worked for three years before getting an MBA at Fordham. He then moved into the internet sports business, first at CBS SportsLine and then at Sports.com, the largest European sports site, where he was based in London. While he was doing well professionally, his alcohol use became increasingly problematic.

In 2001, Gene changed jobs again, becoming chairman and CEO

of a start-up company in San Francisco that provided health-care surgical instrument management and supply tracking software. He asked Tommy to come back to America and work with him. The family missed him. He and Mary and the other kids had visited him in Europe, but they hadn't seen him often, and they were hoping all their kids would eventually come back to California and raise families. So Tommy came back and joined the marketing department of Gene's start-up. It wasn't long before he realized how his son's heavy drinking was affecting his job performance. He moved Tommy to the logistics side of the company, where he fared better. Gene then sold the company and became CEO of a company in Los Angeles, Alteer, which provided software to medical practices. Tommy moved with him.

By then, Tommy was forty and married. His wife, a European woman over a decade younger than he was, began calling Gene, asking for advice regarding Tommy's drinking.

"I would find him in a bar," he recalled, "or passed out in his car in a parking lot. And then I would get him home." Tommy finally agreed to go to rehab, and over the next few years he went to many of the top programs in the country. He began at Betty Ford in Minnesota; he later went to Pathways and Cirque in Utah, and several others.

"Five or six of them, without any success, at tremendous cost," Gene recalled. "Some of these are fifty- or sixty-grand-a-month kinds of places. And none of them took. I would go pick him up at the airport, on his way back from the rehab center, and he was already drunk. He got divorced. He went to a psychiatrist for medication because he was terribly depressed." The psychiatrist helped him get disability payments from Social Security, and he was able to support himself in a small apartment.

But the drinking continued. "It was just one incredible scene after another," he said. "I must have taken him to the ER twenty times. He would be drinking a half gallon of vodka a day, and then as you try to recover from that you go into convulsions. And that's where most alcoholics die—at that stage. And so I kept taking him to the ER. Sometimes if he was bad enough, they'd keep him over. But they'd usually just keep him a few hours, pump liquids into him, and send him home. You don't get much slack when you go to a hospital drunk. They just wanna get you out of there."

Every doctor Tommy saw told him the same thing: if he didn't stop drinking, he would die. And soon.

TOMMY WAS NOT the only medical emergency the family was dealing with. Gretchen was in trouble as well. She and her husband and two daughters had lived in Denver, but after they divorced and he got custody of the kids, she moved to California to be closer to her parents and siblings. Gretchen had a scary auto accident in her past—she was driving her kids home from school when she had flipped her car with them in it. Amazingly, nobody was seriously hurt, but Gretchen was charged with a DUI and forced to go to rehab. So when she got arrested for DUI again, she was given a prison sentence.

Gene talked to Gretchen almost every day—they would practice meditation on the prison phone. He kept her commissary fund stocked so she wouldn't have to live on prison food, and they often had very loving interactions. The same was true for his relationship with Tommy; there were nightmarish moments, but like all medical emergencies, they still brought family members closer. This is one of the fascinating and surprising things about families dealing with these illnesses: it is hard to make people who have never been through it to understand that moments of fear and pain can also bring people together.

In the midst of all this, Gene's wife Mary became ill, suffering from a degenerative lung disease. In early 2016 she went to one of the top hospitals in the country for her illness, which was in Denver, for treatment, and got some relief. While in Denver with his wife, Gene didn't hear from Tommy for a day or two, so he called home for someone to check in on him. Tommy was discovered dead in the bathroom—from what turned out to be multiple organ failure.

Gretchen had to get permission from the prison to attend her brother's funeral.

During this time Gene also became ill and was successfully treated for melanoma. He got more involved with health care and became a board trustee for a major health system in San Diego.

When Gretchen got out of prison, Gene helped set her up in an apartment. But her sobriety was very fragile and her choice of boyfriends less than helpful. She also became more depressed and made several suicide attempts, once by slashing her wrists and twice by stabbing herself in the stomach, leading to brief hospitalizations.

On May 20, 2017, she showed up at her parents' apartment, obviously high, and said she needed to take a shower. Her parents said that would be fine and did not accompany her back to the bedroom. Gretchen stole money and credit cards from their dressers, along with her father's keys, before dashing out and driving away in their car.

Gene called the police. When Gretchen was arrested, she had already spent nearly a thousand dollars of their money. While he considered the possibility that prison might be safer for her, given her condition, Gene did not plan to press charges. He just wanted Gretchen home safe. But because of his and Mary's ages, the police charged her with elder abuse—which, like child endangerment, is a law enforcement priority. She was convicted and sentenced to three years in prison.

Mary Barduson died in February 2018 at the age of seventy-eight. Gretchen had to get a day pass from the Los Colinas Women's Detention Center in Santee—a psychiatric security facility—to attend her mother's funeral. Gretchen's sentence was reduced to a year and a half, and when she was released she and her father doubled down on her treatments. She was able to get into an intensive two-week behavioral health program where she saw a psychiatrist every day, and came out with her first-ever psychiatric diagnosis—after years of primarily being treated in the addiction world.

"The psychiatrist called me toward the end of the program," Gene recalled, "and said, 'The bad news is that Gretchen is bipolar, we are very certain of that. The good news is that we have medication that can really help her.'"

He hoped a psychiatric diagnosis might lead to a turning point in her self-care. "In many medical communities, if you're an alcoholic, then that's *what you are,*" Gene explained. "I've never met an alcoholic anywhere who wouldn't rather be *anything* other than alcoholic. Because then they don't get blamed for it, right?"

Gretchen moved into a new apartment, where Gene had not only delivered her stuff but also some of her late mother's things he thought might help her feel at home—framed pictures, furniture, some of her mom's clothes. They picked up her medication, but she was disappointed to hear that it could be sixty days before it could make her start feeling better. She said she would try to stay on it but immediately complained that the pills made her sleepy.

She was seeing a psychiatrist as well as an alternative medicine therapist. She also participated in a study at the Brain Treatment Center in nearby Carlsbad.

But whenever Gene stopped by her apartment to see how she was doing, there would be an almost empty bottle of vodka on the table in front of her. Sometimes Gretchen needed to be taken to the emergency room because her boyfriend had beaten her up. Then in October 2019, after he hadn't heard from Gretchen for nearly a week, he went to her apartment and let himself in. The place had been trashed, many of the pictures from her mother smashed, with broken glass everywhere. He confronted Gretchen and told her if she didn't stop drinking and trashing the apartment, he could no longer support her.

"Fine," she said, and she started packing.

When her father didn't stop her, she left. Her boyfriend at the time was a drug dealer who had been crashing with her because he didn't have his own place. They went to where he stayed, in a well-established homeless community outside San Diego.

When Gretchen eventually returned to the apartment, she found, to her astonishment, that her father had emptied the place of the rest of her stuff and stopped paying the rent.

She assumed he had just thrown out or given away all of her possessions. "I can't believe he gave everything I own away, all Mom's stuff," she told me when we talked that night. "But, you know, those are my choices. He told me numerous times, 'I'm not gonna sit and watch you die.'"

But, in fact, Gene told me that he still has much of Gretchen's stuff in storage, including her mom's clothes, for when she is sober again.

Until then, she lives outdoors. She has a different boyfriend now—a tall, former high school athlete and veteran who Gene likes because he takes better care of her. They live on his small military pension, SNAP benefits, and they collect bottles and cans from dumpsters and trash cans; they earn twenty to fifty dollars a day turning them in for recycling. They have been trying for a while to qualify for VA housing.

NOT LONG AFTER Gretchen left in 2019, Gene decided he wanted to start a new nonprofit that would bring together everything he knew about medical systems, technology, and substance use to try to fund "a cure for addiction." He called his organization the Addiction Research Institute and has been working hard to launch it—raising $350,000 in initial funding in 2021 and more each year since.

But perhaps the most powerful thing Gene has done to change the world for people struggling with addiction is to allow his family's story to be told, in all its challenging detail. It is a story of pain but also one of courage and resilience. He has been telling it to me unflinchingly, trying to answer every painful question. He wants the world to know how bad addiction and mental illness can get, yet how much is possible as long as the people you love stay alive. And, as a mathematician, computer expert, and an alcoholic in long-term recovery, he is certain he and his organization can make a difference.

In the meantime, he balances a life of enormous extremes. He lives comfortably, near children and grandchildren. He is grateful daily for his sobriety, which has been constant since his twelve-step "birthday" of March 11, 1985, and helps him to "handle many difficult situations and still enjoy life." And yet he is constantly waiting for a phone call, either from Gretchen or *about* Gretchen. She keeps changing cell phones, so he doesn't always know if a call is from her or not.

Sometimes he's relieved if the phone doesn't ring at all.

"I've had so many conversations with the police force," he told me. "If something bad happens, I'll be the first to know. So in a sense, no news is good news. At least she is not in dire shape—if she was, she or someone else would call. And pretty much nothing surprises me anymore."

For several months after he arranged for me to speak to Gretchen, he didn't hear from her at all. Then she called on Mother's Day and asked if he wanted to get together. He doesn't allow her to come to his house anymore, so he went to see her in Santee, in a little park near the Walmart parking lot. They met at the benches there.

As she approached, he was relieved to see that she was no longer wheelchair-bound, but her walking was still badly impaired. She was pushing her wheelchair, using it as a walker. She sat down and they talked.

"She was sober on Mother's Day, and we had a good talk," he said. "She told me, 'I'm gonna stop this, Dad, and get a job.' I said, 'Well, you have a big advantage over most people on the street. You have an education, you've got a great personality, you're pretty, and you have a record of doing great work on the job.' She said, 'I know, I know.'"

He dared, again, as he always will, to hope. And then he didn't hear from her for more than six weeks. When she called, she was clearly drunk and said she had been drunk pretty much the entire time since he had seen her last. She asked if he might consider getting her a motel room for a night or two. She said she hadn't had a shower in forty days.

He arranged for a room on a Sunday night in mid-July. Since I had been trying to arrange a follow-up conversation with Gretchen for months, Gene texted the next morning to let me know she was at the motel, with her boyfriend, and this would be a good time for us to talk before her 11:00 A.M. checkout. I reached out to her by text, as did Gene, but she didn't call. He offered to let them stay another night and then arranged for us to talk that next morning. The time was all arranged, and I got a text from Gene at 10:25 A.M. saying, "She just texted me and she can talk now." But when I called, there was no answer. I sent her a Zoom link and Gene texted her to click on it and join, but she didn't. A few minutes later, he texted and said she wasn't responding to his texts either.

"I'm afraid she is in a really bad place right now," he wrote. We rescheduled for an hour later. At that time, he texted, "I called her room, talked to her boyfriend . . . she is in the shower, will be able to talk in a few minutes." A second later he texted, "BF said she has been sick . . . a little vodka flu I suspect."

Ten minutes later, he texted, "She will call me in a few minutes . . . she is struggling with a hangover . . . BF says she will be on zoom in a few minutes."

Then neither of us heard from her or the boyfriend again, and when Gene inquired at the motel, they had checked out.

I later called Gene, just to tell him I understood, in some small way, what he goes through.

"At some point, she will sober up," he told me. "And, the truth is, I don't have the same anxiety I used to have about this. Even during the last couple of years of Tommy's life, when he was drinking heavily, we had some good times. I stopped trying to fix him. And these things like Gretchen's irresponsibility? At some level they just remind me of what an asshole I was, when that was *me* drinking. So, I'm getting better at handling that."

He said he got an email the other day from a woman who was helping with the fundraising for his new addiction research institute. She had been sending out videos of people sharing brief, powerful versions of their stories.

"How do you handle all this?" she asked him. "It's all so sad."

He told her, "I'm not sad all the time."

Chapter Eleven

Aidan

Aidan Understein was already well into his junior year at Appalachian State University in North Carolina before everyone found out what he had been hiding.

It happened during the reception of his younger sister's bat mitzvah in Chapel Hill, where he had grown up. A handsomely nerdy twenty-year-old, with thick eyebrows and full grinning lips, he had managed to keep his eyes open and remain seated upright through the ceremony. But at a certain point during the reception, he lost consciousness—and his face fell into his plate.

He was quickly removed from the reception room, and when he regained consciousness, his grandmother volunteered to take him back to the house. Later, when his parents got home, Aidan didn't say much about what could have caused him to pass out. But it turned out his parents had another possible source of information.

Several days earlier, they had made him get a hair-follicle drug test because they were concerned that he might be using something. In the hustle and bustle of the bat mitzvah weekend, they hadn't yet checked the Labcorp website for the results. And when they did, they were stunned. They had expected a positive result for something, but not for so many drugs, including crack cocaine; the opiates hydromorphone (Dilaudid), morphine, and codeine; as well as two medication-assisted treatment (MAT) drugs used to treat opiate addiction (which can also be abused to get high), methadone and buprenorphine (Suboxone). Had he been tested several months earlier, he would have been positive for heroin as well.

"I finally realized what I had developed into," he told me. "I was always in denial of the possibility . . . that I could be, y'know, a full-blown opiate addict."

His parents and grandparents were beside themselves, especially because they were quite knowledgeable about mental illness and addiction. His mother was in recovery. His maternal grandmother, who lived near them, was in recovery. And his maternal grandfather was a nationally known, UCLA-trained psychiatrist and health-care executive, Dr. Murray Zucker, who was then a senior medical director for the behavioral health division of the country's largest health insurer (and a friend of mine, which is how I met the And Understeins).

The family had always known that Aidan, the oldest of their three kids, was a little "different," suffered from some social anxiety and ADHD, perhaps was "on the spectrum," and had been impacted by challenges in his parents' marriage. But that described a lot of kids his age.

What they didn't know was the extent of his complex and dangerous secret life, buying and selling various drugs on the Dark Web from people all over the world, using thousands of dollars' worth of every conceivable kind of currency.

As Aidan explained to me his vast experience with the Dark Web drug business—having boxes and packages from all over the world delivered to his college postal box—I was shocked. I am no longer amazed by how much any person can drink or ingest; I have been there myself and have heard too many stories from people I care about. But I must admit, I had never heard anything like Aidan's saga of his online drug trade—both the incredible risks he took with seriously scary people and the amazing amount he had learned about chemistry and pharmacology, not so much to improve his health but to improve his business.

"In addition to the dark underworld that Aidan thought was just a game," Murray told me, shaking his head in disbelief, "he also got to be, or at least he fancied himself to be, a psychopharmacology expert. After we found out about all this, he would enjoy discussions with me about neurotransmitters and all the latest findings. He was pretty up on the literature. It was kind of bizarre having a conversation about this with him. But I thought, Wow, you know, he really can get into a subject in depth. Maybe he has a future in pharmacy work and I should steer him in that direction."

He thought for a second. "Of course," he added, "that would be very dangerous."

By the time I got to meet Aidan, he was twenty-eight. He had left college and had been to well-known rehabs, clinics, wilderness programs, and sober living environments all over the country, many times over. He had been to enough facilities that he could compare and contrast treatment modalities, staffing, even the differences between West Coast and East Coast addiction care sensibilities.

Yet, he had ended up at a place hardly anyone had heard of, not far from where Amy and I live in South Jersey, a "structured sober living" community called Surfside Recovery in Ventnor City. And everyone who knew him said they had never been so optimistic before about his chances to finally have a sustained recovery—and a life.

AIDAN WAS BORN in Rockville, Maryland, in 1995. His mother, Timna, had grown up in the west, with parents who were ex-hippies, before getting a master's in education from Columbia and becoming a teacher; his father, Jamie, helped run a specialized employment agency just for dentists and dental technicians. Aidan had a younger brother and then a sister, before the family decided in 2003 to move to North Carolina, where Timna's mother had settled after her divorce (while her father, Murray, remained in California).

From the time Aidan was six, he recalled "feeling empty-ish" at certain times of the year. "I thought it was pretty normal," he said. "I thought that, like, every winter, everybody felt soulless." He later recognized that he was experiencing what is referred to as "seasonal depression." He felt a certain sense of detachment. His hobbies, even his beloved Matchbox cars, "became less of hobbies and more like chores." And it seemed as if every year after that, whatever sport or club he signed up for, he would quit when winter hit. He recalled his parents being okay with that.

"They were very hands-off," he recalled. "My mom was definitely a helicopter parent, but without the authoritarian aspect. So, there was never a scolding or a punishment."

The first sign he had an addictive predisposition occurred when he was eleven and he became obsessed with playing the new online, multiplayer fantasy game *RuneScape*.

"I would wake up at five A.M. to play it," he explained. "But if you tried to wake me up at five A.M. to go to school or do a chore, fat chance."

His parents had communication issues from the beginning, but their lives and marriage became more challenged when Aidan was twelve. His mom was diagnosed with melanoma on the bottom of her foot, and after the surgery she became obsessed about mole checking (which did not spare her several additional melanomas and surgeries). She also started drinking more; it wasn't the first time—she had struggled with alcohol use since she was a teen, as had her mother and grandmother.

That same year of his mother's skin cancer diagnosis, Aidan was diagnosed with ADHD. His pediatrician tried to get him to take the stimulant dexmethylphenidate (Focalin), but the first dose made him too buzzy: "I remember being at Target with my mom, zooming around the store and talking to all the cashiers." He tried one more dose on a school day and then, "I realized it just wasn't for me." Later, he tried other types of stimulants but used them more situationally, usually only on days when he felt he needed help to succeed on a test—when he had a midterm, or was taking the PSAT.

The following year there was more family trauma. In September 2008, Aidan's eighty-four-year-old great-grandfather, Irv Shuman, who he had seen just a few months before at his own bar mitzvah, was murdered in Phoenix. A legendary real estate developer and philanthropist in the Jewish community, Irv had been very active in Republican politics in Arizona. (He was a good friend of our own family friend, Senator John McCain.) Shuman was found beaten and strangled in his office in central Phoenix, which devastated the family. His gold Lexus was stolen, turning up in San Bernadino, California, several days later, but his murder became one of Arizona's best-known unsolved crimes.

The only good thing to come of this was that Aidan, like all of Shuman's grandchildren, was left a trust fund. Nobody could have guessed how much of the money he would need for mental health and addiction treatment.

When Aidan was fifteen, his parents sent him to a psychotherapist to help with anxiety. So he had someone to talk to when, out of nowhere, he experienced his first panic attack while camping with friends in the woods one night.

"I remember feeling like I was going to throw up and then all of a sudden hitting the ground," he said. "I didn't know. Was this a seizure? Was it a heart attack? I just didn't know. After a few minutes it stopped. Later, the therapist explained that panic attacks aren't deadly, they go away."

He didn't tell the therapist that, besides weed, he was now drinking, taking hydrocodone (Vicodin), and using cocaine. He also didn't tell anyone how he was paying for it. Not long after his bar mitzvah, he somehow figured out how to create a PayPal account tied to his personal savings account without his parents realizing. When packages started arriving for him at the house from eBay, his parents were surprised but they didn't pry.

"Once, when my friends and I were into making home movies," he told me, "I wanted to buy prop cap guns for it. So I ordered four 'lots,' but, I didn't really know what 'a lot' was. So 250 cap guns arrive at the door. My parents were at a loss to understand this, but I don't remember getting scolded or disciplined."

His strategy was to tell his parents just enough that they thought he was being honest with them. "So I kept everything except weed and alcohol from them," he said. "I figured if I divulged enough, then it would seem plausible that's all that was happening."

This worked until they found Vicodin pills in his closet. "My parents sat me down," he recalled. "They started the conversation 'What's wrong? What is so wrong that you need to take these things?'"

But, finally, his mother asked, "Do you know what happens to people who take these? You'll become a heroin addict."

Aidan told her, "That's not true at all."

"I wish it wasn't," she shot back. And then she told him, for the first time, a little bit about her experience in twelve-step meetings for her own addiction to alcohol. This was a really big deal for his mother, to share about her own recovery. But, it did not, at the time, impress Aidan.

"My mom was like, 'Listen, I'm part of a program where, you know, alcoholics get together,' whatever, blah, blah, blah," he said. "She said she had a few friends who started with Vicodin 'and now they're heroin addicts. And if I kept on this path . . .'"

In fact, he recalled the conversation mostly because of the irony of a situation that unfolded not long after. It turned out that one of his heroin dealers was someone his mom had sponsored.

None of this made much impact on Aidan at the time. He was surprised by how often he did not get into real trouble. "One time I came home drunk, very drunk," he recalled, "and they came in my room in the morning and were, like, 'Oh, my God, you were so drunk last night that *you're still intoxicated right now*. And your car is here, which means that *you drove home drunk*.' And instead of being, you know, grounded forever, my punishment was that over the weekend, I would have to apply to ten more colleges—and I couldn't drive for a week. And I got my car keys back in a couple of days anyway."

The only time he remembered getting "super, super in trouble" was after a family vacation to Costa Rica. "I bought out like an entire pharmacy of Tylenol with codeine," he explained. "And other parents found some text messages between me and my friend about it. In Costa Rica, they sell meds by the day, because a lot of people are day laborers and don't have enough money to buy thirty days' worth at a time. So I went to a pharmacy and asked for 'codina.' And they said, 'How many?' And I thought that meant, 'How many boxes?' so I said, 'Two,' and they brought out two tablets. That's when I realized that I could ask for a lot more. I bought like five hundred tablets. I paid fifty American dollars. And I used them all."

This was the first time he realized what a tolerance he had developed to opioids. "I had to crush up the tablets to get the amount necessary to get me high," he recalled. But he didn't think of it as "getting high." It was more that "Once I took an opioid, I felt normal. To the extent that a normal person could derive pleasure out of, say, a stimulant, I couldn't—it would just add to my anxiety. But when I took an opioid, I felt like I could actually enter life and enjoy what normal people might be able to enjoy."

Once he started doing stronger drugs, he smoked pot less often and only drank if he was going out for the whole weekend. "So, in my parents' eyes, things were actually *looking* better," he recalled. "Because when I was smoking pot and drinking a lot, I didn't care about things. But when I was doing opioids and ADHD meds and cocaine, my grades went up. My aspirations for life suddenly appeared. And I started taking honors courses and AP courses, things that would, on paper, present as someone who was caring about their life."

However, Aidan nearly failed to graduate from high school because he had been absent more than the maximum allowable thirty days. But his psychologist wrote a note saying many of those days were medical issues, which allowed him to finish. At the time, Aidan saw this as a way to game the system. Only much later did he realize how right the psychologist had been about his medical issues.

BY THE TIME he got to college at Appalachian State—about two and a half hours west of Chapel Hill, in Boone—Aidan had figured out how to do more than just use PayPal to buy drugs.

"'The first place I learned about was Silk Road, on the Deep Web, one of the first black-market sites, and you could get pretty much anything you wanted," he explained. He learned how to make payments from an online tutorial that explained "how to link a bank to a cryptocurrency website that transfers to and from a crypto wallet."

He had everything delivered to the post office box for his dorm room. "So, this is where everything took off," he said. "I was ordering different kinds of heroin. I was ordering different grades or tiers of cocaine. I was ordering methamphetamine. I was ordering pills from pharmaceutical factories in Pakistan, in Iraq. Everything was coming in all at once."

While he was using all these drugs at the time, Aidan thought of his Dark Web activities mostly as a business. However, his grandfather, Murray, told me he thought it was mostly just "a game" to Aidan.

"I was mortified when I found out the extent of his involvement," he said. "But when he did start telling us about it, he would be very forthright in describing it, as if he was talking about a *baseball game* or something. But he was talking about being involved with people who could *kill him*. To this day, I'm not sure how much of this was 'spectrum' kind of lack of judgment and how much was being involved with drugs and how it affects your thinking. But his judgment was very poor."

Aidan had a girlfriend since his last years of high school, who had been worried about his increasing drug use but stayed with him. When she realized during his freshman year in college just how far it had all escalated—not only in terms of the volume of his use but the recklessness of all the things he was trying—she said she needed a break.

"I would slowly just break more and more boundaries," he recalled. "But it was also just too hard. I remember she told me that, for years, when I said to her I was feeling depressed, or feeling anxious, she heard the words come out of my mouth but didn't understand the feelings; she had never felt them herself. But, she said, 'Now I do.' So, being with me doing drugs was so draining and sad that she now knew what depression felt like. I remember feeling very sad about the breakup but, actually, happy for her, if that makes any sense. She was protecting herself."

By the time he was twenty, and a junior in college, Aidan was in a fraternity, "so it was even easier to meet people" and business was expanding.

"I opened up a new account at Wells Fargo and I was establishing a credit line," he explained. "So, the good part was that there was always leftover currency to purchase drugs that I needed. The bad part was that I started getting physically dependent and began purchasing heavier things. Fentanyl was just coming out at that point—it was still a luxury and not yet a deadly finished product. So everything that I purchased online became heavier duty, higher quantities. I had a safe in my room with hundreds of sedatives. The safe had a timer, and I would try to control my use by setting a time limit. I would take a few pills out of the safe, and then set it not to open again for six hours."

Aidan was partying more, "and I guess I was pretty promiscuous. I didn't feel like a real person unless I was on opioids. And it all came to a head because it was twenty bucks a tablet and I needed one every two or three hours, on top of the cocaine to keep me awake, which is like eighty bucks, so it came out to three or four hundred dollars a day. It was unsustainable. And so, when it was really a sinking ship, I started to drink heavily to try to mask symptoms of withdrawal. And that would just make it worse."

Then his face fell into his food at the bat mitzvah.

After that incident, he actually convinced his parents they should let him return to college, since he only had a few weeks left. He decided when he got there that he would detox by himself. He gave away many of his drugs and flushed the opiates down the toilet. "And the next day I began cold turkey detox," he recalled. "It was awful. It was hellish. And because I did it cold turkey, it messed me up longer than it should have."

Within months, Aidan had withdrawn from college. His mother also left his father, so Aidan was moving back and forth between their homes. His mother forced Aidan to attend an intensive outpatient program at ASAP, the Alcohol and Substance Abuse Program at the University of North Carolina at Chapel Hill. It was his first serious treatment for substance use disorder, but he didn't take it very seriously.

"To me it was just like group therapy," he said. "I met a councilman there who had a DUI and needed to appease the public. There were a lot of high school kids that got caught doing coke."

When he finished the outpatient program, his parents said that if they caught him using any drug or drinking, he would be sent to rehab. That scared him because he didn't really know what rehab was. "I was thinking it would be like being sent to a homeless shelter," he said.

He was seeing a psychiatrist and working in a grocery store where they did random saliva tests. He started using heroin and cocaine and predictably got a positive drug test. Within weeks, in April 2016, he was sent away for a ninety-day inpatient rehab at one of the fanciest substance use hospitals in the country, Cirque Lodge in Utah.

It was the first time he ever went through detox and then a

comprehensive differential diagnosis. His mother and his grandfather—who knew one of his treating physicians—tried to impress upon Cirque Lodge that Aidan was unique because he had an undiagnosed autism spectrum disorder.

Murray explained to me that in substance use treatment and recovery groups, the issue of how an underlying intellectual or developmental disability (IDD) can and should impact care is still not taken seriously enough.

"With someone like Aidan, his social skills are very good, so he is able to convince people he is okay and doesn't have these 'spectrum' kinds of issues," he said. "It also, strangely, makes people overestimate his IQ, which is a strength of his, in a way, but also gets him in trouble because therapists expect a lot more of him than they should. It's easy for an evaluation to miss the unique social difficulties and cognitive aspects."

I asked Murray what the differences should be in treating someone with a spectrum disorder for addiction.

"In most cases, patients get treated with essentially a one-size-fits-all approach—which is a general problem in all mental health and addiction care," he said. "If you treat someone like Aidan in the typical way, he's going to feel more out of place than other people, and that standard recovery approach just isn't gonna work. If you did adjust for it, the therapist would take a different approach to education, to feedback and reward, with maybe fewer expectations that would be difficult to fulfill. I'm not necessarily talking about dumbing down the treatment, just making it more particular to that person's weaknesses and strengths."

These are just some of the underlying challenges in Aidan's struggle to remain sober and healthy. And it has been an epic battle with addiction.

During the next eight years, Aidan would have twenty-three different forms of extended care: repeated inpatient hospitalizations for a month or more, stays in sober living communities, in some cases up to a year, a three-month experiential outdoors program, and quite a few emergency room visits for overdoses, followed by short detoxes. In 2016 alone, he spent ninety days inpatient at Cirque, followed by a month in the young adult sober living community Balance House (also in Utah), then back to Cirque for another thirty days inpatient, after which he moved to Southern California for a sober living/intensive outpatient program at PCH (Psychological Care and Healing) Center in Los Angeles, then sober living at Casa Vista in Venice, California.

There he not only started doing heroin again but also began abusing the antidiarrheal drug Imodium. "I realized if you take seventy or a hundred of them, it's pretty similar to an opioid high," he said. "I became adept at taking thirty or forty of those small teal tablets at a time with a large sip of Pepsi. But the withdrawals were worse than any opioid I've ever done."

At the beginning of 2017, Aidan moved to the Sober College addiction treatment center in L.A. After several months, he started using again. And in August he overdosed on fentanyl but was revived in time. After recovering, he was allowed to continue in the program.

During that year he also lost one of his closest friends, Eric, who was also in and out of recovery. They were both still in the program but living in apartments off the grounds. One day, Eric texted him and asked if he was still sober.

"I had been through this enough times," he explained, "to know that when you ask someone that, it's because you're hoping they will say 'no' and you can go over to their house and drink and use with them. I kind of knew he was fishing. So I lied and said I was still sober. We texted a little bit more about life, and then that was it. The next morning I was in bed with my girlfriend and I got a call from our old counselor in the program. He said, 'Eric is dead.' I actually assumed it was some sick joke he was playing on me, and I remember laughing hysterically at first. At that time, it was more plausible to me that a substance abuse therapist would tell me a joke about a dead best friend. And then I cried for a week straight."

After that, Aidan remained sober for a few months. Then he overdosed again and was sent back to Utah for detox at the University of Utah hospital and a sixty-day inpatient stay at Recovery Ways, a rehab hospital in Salt Lake City.

He then came home to North Carolina, staying in a sober living intensive outpatient program at Midtown Recovery. "I was working in a restaurant," he recalled, "and doing a lot of cocaine, even though I was on Suboxone maintenance." (Suboxone—a combination of buprenorphine and naloxone—only helps prevent relapse on opiates; there is no Suboxone equivalent for cocaine and stimulants.)

"It was ridiculous, me trying to juggle maintenance, recreational drug use, and the job," he said, "and it ended on November 26, 2019, with my parents holding a private intervention, just the two of them with my grandpa on the phone. And I eventually agreed to go back to Utah and detox off the Suboxone. And then I went to a wilderness program."

THERE ARE MANY types of wilderness experiences available across the country—with varying degrees of interest in medical or psychological treatment. Aidan's family chose the Elements Traverse Wilderness Therapy Treatment for Young Adults, which was in the middle of Utah, in Huntington. Like all wilderness programs, it included a lot of team and resiliency building through outdoor living. But it also had a strong focus on talk therapy, specifically dialectical behavioral therapy (DBT). DBT is a therapy that grew out of short-term, directed cognitive behavioral therapy, but added aspects of mindfulness training, emotional regulation, and distress tolerance, in part to try to improve how CBT worked with patients who were frequently suicidal. (It is also viewed as more feminist and gender-inclusive, and more concerned with spirituality, than CBT; it was invented by a female psychology researcher, Marsha Linehan.)

Aidan considered this combination of wilderness and DBT as the first truly "life-changing experience" he ever had in treatment.

"I always saw wilderness as the scariest option," he said. "It always seemed like a last resort, like boot camp. But this was . . . well, I wish it had been the first resort. I went through a paradigm shift of every single category; a psychic change occurred there.

"You wake up when they tell you to wake up. And if they say, 'Break down camp and pack up, we're getting back on trail in an hour,' then you do that. And you hike all day. Everything that you live off of is built up and broken down by you and your companions. It's up to you to uphold the law of the land. If you don't particularly like someone doing something, then it's up to the group to uphold that standard. So it really builds leadership, it builds responsibility and accountability, from hearing feedback, taking feedback, implementing feedback. And I liked the DBT model. Everything good in my life after that, I credit to them. Anytime I've ever been able to hold down recovery, hold down any kind of clean time, hold down any job, hold down any college courses, or lived on my own successfully, even for a brief period—all of that is from wilderness therapy."

Aidan lived outdoors with his Elements Traverse counselors and fellow patients for over three months. When he finished, he felt like a new person. To maintain his sobriety, he was sent to a sober community in Tucson, In Balance, to live in its collegiate transition program. Unfortunately, he graduated from Elements Traverse on March 9, 2020—two days before the World Health Organization declared COVID a pandemic. So he spent his time at In Balance—including his twenty-fifth birthday—in lockdown.

Without much access to the outside world, he stayed sober there for eight months. He took classes at the University of Arizona and did well. When people started going out, "we started going out partying sober," he recalled. "I was having a great time, going dancing, clubbing, walking around the city late at night, just having fun. I was FaceTiming with my mom and grandma every morning. It was pristine, the way I was living. It was beyond clean, and one of the first times that the promises of twelve-step were coming through."

Graduates of that program can then transition to living independently while still remaining in outpatient treatment at In Balance. They also have a graduation ceremony, which family members watched remotely because of COVID. Aidan's speech was mostly about how wilderness treatment had changed his life and given him his first useful tools to address challenges.

"Aidan gave a speech I couldn't believe," Murray told me. "He was so articulate and so proud and so thankful and it was a beautiful thing. He had been camping during the winter in Utah, out by himself going through all this rigorous stuff, hanging by his nails on a cliff, to survive or not. The approach was really do-or-die and he loved it. He opened up and learned he could be self-reliant.

"I just wanted to hit the pause button and say, 'Okay, now that's you forever.' Unfortunately, it wasn't."

IT WASN'T LONG before Aidan slipped.

After moving into a Tucson apartment, "I decided to start looking at the Dark Web again, just to see if it was still there," he said. "Of course, it was, better than ever."

He ordered a gram of heroin. "I got it, I sniffed one line of it, and I freaked out," he recalled. "I threw the rest of it away. But then I started thinking maybe that was worse than if I had done the whole bag. Because now in the back of my head, I had a lie: if you can do one line of heroin and then throw out the rest, then you could probably do it again and be fine. So that delusion started creeping back in.

"It's never *just* a slipup. That's unfortunately not how it works for an addict like me."

Soon, he was online looking for something that wouldn't technically violate his sobriety but could get him high. He selected the drug Fioricet, a headache medicine that contains acetaminophen (Tylenol) and caffeine but also a barbiturate, butalbital, which he learned from researching wasn't then federally scheduled as being very addictive by the DEA, although different states had different rules about it. (The ingredient, used in the old-school benzodiazepine, is Schedule IV—the more addictive drugs, which are also more restricted, are Schedule I, II, and III.) He found an online doctor who would write the prescription, and soon he couldn't get enough. So he explored buying an alternative version of its active ingredient on eBay—by ordering what is called "new old stock," antique but unopened medications people generally use for old-time drugstore displays and collectibles.

"I started buying sealed vials of barbiturates from the sixties, seventies, and eighties," he explained. "So I was very bad off, dumbfounded at how quickly things had gone wrong with my life."

He eventually started using heroin and cocaine again and selling from the Dark Web to pay for his own drugs. He spent much of 2021 spiraling farther down in Tucson.

"I got to the point where my tolerance was very high," he recalled, "and then heroin started to disappear, and no one had it. And I was wondering why till a friend of mine told me people weren't even doing heroin anymore. They were smoking fentanyl, which was delivered as synthetic oxycodone tablets. I remember buying a few of those and realizing that even though they aren't very 'recreational' in terms of how high they make you, they were required once you hit a certain level of tolerance. At that point, it was either quit entirely or continue on and upgrade to fentanyl—which is what I did."

Everything about his life and drugs suddenly became more dangerous. "I was running around with a gun," he recalled, incredulous. "It was a Glock 43X special I got from a friend. I never actually shot it or got shot at. But I saw gun violence, and it's more the constant threat that gets to you. Because in Tucson, if you hear a gunshot, that's normal. But if you don't hear it and someone's close to you with a gun, that's honestly scarier. Twice I had someone put a gun to my head. I'm not proud of that. I was involved with people who I *never* want to be involved with. I didn't trust anything or anyone because I had cocaine-induced paranoia. And it was all just terrible. Everything was, like, just one gigantic, cold sweat nightmare."

SOME FAMILY MEMBERS were beginning to run out of patience and sympathy for Aidan. During a particularly intense part of our conversation, his grandfather, Murray, admitted he was one of them.

"I would say my involvement, and don't print this, has been variable," he said. "At times I'm preoccupied and it's too frustrating. Part of it is that sometimes when I was with him, I knew Aidan was just jabbering away and it was all bullshit. And that was very hard for me. I mean, if someone's paying me five hundred an hour to do that, okay, fine. But, when it's my own grandson, you know, I must admit at times I just got worn down. It's like, I don't wanna hear it: enough, *enough*."

I stopped him and asked if he would consider changing his mind about not printing what he had said. It was pretty honest, I explained, and he was hardly the only person in the world who had thought that way.

He said it would be okay. "As I'm hearing myself say that, I'm not particularly proud of myself as a grandfather," he said. "But I do think it's common, human, and normal. And I think it would be important for the public to hear that even a professional can get worn down and tired trying to help."

He said there was another aspect of family involvement people rarely talked about. "There were discussions about whether or not to invite Aidan to a family get-together," he said, "and I mean occasions he had *always* attended before, like Thanksgiving. Because there were so many family gatherings that were disappointing or uncomfortable because Aidan was acting weird, and people were saying, 'He's probably on drugs.' There were times during planning occasions when some family members said, 'If he's going to be there, I'm not coming and I'm not bringing my kids.'"

It upset Murray to hear himself say all this. "This is such a sad aspect of the dynamic of recovery," he said. "The person becomes the black sheep, becomes toxic, to the very people he needs most to be a comforting, understanding, reassuring family. They just get burned out."

I told him I knew exactly what he was talking about. I had been through it myself during many of those same years—teens and twenties—when Aidan was experiencing it. When my dad would say to my brother, "All Patrick needs is a good swift kick in the ass." And my mother, during the many recurrences of her lifelong alcohol use disorder, was also sometimes treated dismissively—especially when her drinking was the most socially or politically inconvenient. We were not always as kind as we could and should have been.

I remember going to McLean Hospital for the one family meeting when she was being treated there, and the therapist asked, "How do you feel?" And my sister, who was generally very mild-mannered and easy-peasy, said, "I don't care if my mother dies." I just remember that so clearly, because she voiced the rage of having to deal with people who suffer from these illnesses and it went right to the heart of the big problem we have—which is getting any kind of political power behind advocacy when families are so burned out.

I told Murray I had recently watched a family member go through eating disorder treatment and was amazed at how much family-based therapy there was to teach people how to be good family peers. It wasn't just that one forced family meeting at the hospital. It's about teaching the family in an ongoing way but also letting them vent and understand that their feelings are normal and natural. It's considered the gold standard of care for eating disorders but still isn't something everyone knows is available, so it's less commonly used for other mental illnesses and substance use disorders.

Murray agreed. "You can write a Suboxone prescription and that'll work for some people. But without addressing these family issues . . ."

One day, something his mother texted him, almost in passing, really resonated with Aidan.

He looked down at his phone. "It's getting worse and u know it," he read.

And, for some reason, for the very first time, he didn't obfuscate or offer some overly intellectual reason why she was wrong. He simply told her the truth.

"It is I know," he texted back.

He realized his addiction was "like a cancer that's getting worse. I was either going to decide to die from it, or go get treatment for it. And I thought, 'Screw it, I'm doing it.'"

Just as he was turning twenty-seven in the spring of 2022, he signed up for a detox program in Tucson called Cottonwood. He stayed there for a month, and for the first time was prescribed—among other meds—a maintenance dose of naltrexone (Vivitrol), which took away his cravings for drugs. Previously he had only ever used Suboxone, which replaces some of the feelings created by opiates. He had always refused naltrexone before because, intellectually, he disagreed with the idea of taking away feelings. But he realized that he no longer had the luxury of such intellectual disagreements.

He moved back East, and in May he checked into a structured sober living program in Washington, D.C., called The Palisades House. He had five sober months of living there—all except for one twenty-hour period in August that started out as an evening stroll before curfew and ended in a B-movie nightmare. Ostensibly because his roommate's snoring was getting worse and he was having trouble filling his prescription for the sleep aid zolpidem (Ambien)—but, as is true for so many with substance use disorders, it's always "ostensibly" something—he managed to find a doctor in Arizona who would call in a prescription to D.C. for twelve of the barbiturate headache pills he had used to dodge drug tests before. He told his counselor he was out for a walk at ten-thirty and would be back soon, got the pills, took them all, and just kept walking. He ended up at a motel where a dealer sold him every kind of drug he had been avoiding; he used them there in the dealer's room—even though the naltrexone blocked some of them—and woke up the next morning with the dealer and a prostitute sleeping nearby.

At first, he was convinced the whole thing must have been a nightmare. When he started vomiting profusely, he realized it wasn't.

While he was gone, the facility alerted his family that he was missing. His mother and stepfather combed the city's emergency rooms, morgues, and back alleys for hours, convinced he had overdosed and died. He finally made his way back to the facility, throwing up periodically. When he returned, he was so ill and freaked out that they gave him another chance and let him stay.

Several months later, he left the residential part of the program and moved into an Airbnb on Dupont Circle with a girlfriend. He continued working with a sober coach in the program and getting drug tested weekly; naltrexone was effectively controlling his cravings.

But, around Thanksgiving, he fell into what his mother described as "the most rapid decline I had seen . . . a new level of sick." He looked so terrible and was acting so strangely at the family Thanksgiving dinner that when the weekend was over and she took her other two children to say goodbye to Aidan at his apartment before they flew home, she thought, "This could be the last time they ever see him."

What she didn't know was that he had not renewed his prescription for naltrexone, unbalancing his drug cocktail and making his ADHD medicine much stronger. He relapsed again, including a full week during which he remembered doing nothing but cocaine until his nostrils were bloody and screamingly painful and he was completely disoriented. His mother found him this way, called the police, and tried to get him committed for medical care. While he was at the hospital, his mother and stepfather packed up all his possessions and loaded them into the car. Unfortunately, the hospital wouldn't hold him and sent him home while they were finishing up the packing. He refused to go home with them, so he sat in the apartment for three full days over Christmas, with none of his stuff except for his cell phone (so he could order pizza).

"I was hit with the ultimatum: go to treatment or be homeless," he said. He chose treatment. This time, he went to the Recovery Centers of America (RCA) facility in Waldorf, Maryland.

"Needing rehab after doing drugs for only a week humbled me a lot," he said. "It was the learning experience that showed me that not only have I been addicted to drugs, but I carry the symptoms of substance use disorder in *everything I do.* It was the first time I ever truly understood that and internalized that I had always lived life that way."

The RCA facility wasn't as luxurious and exclusive as other places he had been. And that was a good thing. "It was extremely humbling," he said. "I wasn't treating it like a hotel, like all the other places. This was like, I need to refocus *everything* and truly reprioritize *everything.* I mean, I gave up not only my phone but my *phone number,* so I couldn't contact people and they couldn't find me. I gave up my laptop. I was like, I'm done with everything that's connected me to the past that eventually sucks me back in."

While there, he and his family talked to his caregivers about what Aidan really needed to succeed. They recommended a much more long-term experience, but something different than what he had tried before. The family chose a place pretty far off their radar of well-known facilities: Surfside Recovery, in Ventnor City, New Jersey, an innovative sober living community for men ages seventeen to thirty-five. It was much more structured, restrictive, and interactive than normal sober living—which is usually a group residence with regular twelve-step meetings, but with a certain amount of freedom to work in the outside world. Surfside is a residential program, but it has more of the in-your-face intensity associated with several hours a day spent at a really good intensive outpatient program. It also offers different phases of treatment and oversight—paying close attention to everything from what you say in group therapy to where you are on your checklist of making amends. And there is an emphasis on physical activity, which reminded Aidan of his successful wilderness training—although it was much more New Jersey than Utah. (One of the outdoor activities was cleaning the pens at the Funny Farm Rescue and Sanctuary, which takes in animals of all sizes that have been abused, neglected, or abandoned.)

When I met Aidan, he had been at Surfside for over four months and was still in Phase 1, which is called "Rebuild." He wasn't sure when he would move to the next phase. The program follows each patient's progress individually—everything from finishing the first five of the twelve steps with a sponsor, to doing community service, taking care of your own room and cooking meals, preparing resumes, and writing "family letters" to those you have hurt. You also don't move on until "sneaky and manipulative behavior has ended."

The next time we spoke, he was in Phase 2, "Rediscover," and had moved to the "second house," which is smaller, and you only have one roommate rather than several. Phase 2 includes exploring personal objectives and writing cover letters but also focuses on steps six through nine of the twelve steps, including the process of making amends.

Phase 2, so far, had been emotionally tumultuous for Aidan. In the first weeks, one of his roommates from Phase 1, Nick, was found in a car, dead from an overdose of fentanyl. He was twenty-nine, just a little older than Aidan.

I asked how the death had impacted him.

"I got really sad because he was one of my best friends," he explained. "But it's all the same level of sadness to me because, well, how would I put this . . . after the fourth or fifth person you lose, you start to realize it's not normal to invest your emotions in someone else. There is camaraderie and brotherly love in the program for sure. But I can't have prolonged sadness over someone's choice, no matter the consequences, because at the end of the day it's free will.

"To make it in recovery, I have to invest in myself, so that I can be there for others. I'm not going to invest in someone else so they can be there for me. I don't want to sound cynical, because I'm not. But the gift of sobriety is self-sufficiency."

He turned away for a moment. "It's not so much that I don't trust anybody else," he said. "It's just that I want to get to a place where I can trust myself."

As difficult as the loss of his friend had been, Aidan was emotionally buoyed several weeks later when he went to Washington, D.C., for his "amends trip." Phase 2 requires Surfside patients to complete at least their first ten "amends," so they are encouraged to organize a short trip that will allow them to meet multiple people in their lives in a short time. His mother deemed the concept "fucking brilliant" and didn't understand why, in all her years in AA and her years taking Aidan to programs, she had never heard of such a thing before.

The highlight of her "amends trip" interaction with Aidan was the Thursday afternoon that they attended an AA meeting together, along with Aidan's grandmother, sitting next to each other in a circle of chairs and sharing from the heart. He told the group he was there "to make amends to my mom and my nana" and when he pointed to them, the whole room burst into tears.

Aidan told me the highlight for him, however, was a much less predictable meeting with his childhood best friend, Ben, who he had known pretty much since birth. Their mothers were still friends, but Aidan and Ben hadn't seen or spoken to each other for nearly a decade.

"As I went down the drug addiction path," Aidan told me, "I just felt we were in such different worlds. I never talked to him because he's so normal, and I didn't want to bring any of my shit into such an innocent world." He wasn't even sure Ben would speak to him.

They went for coffee in Adams Morgan. "Within five minutes, it was just like no time had passed; the connection was back," he recalled, with a big smile. "It turns out he's been following me, through our moms talking, *the whole time*. He said, 'I've literally been keeping up with your story like it's, you know, fucking *news,* the headline of the week!'"

Aidan told him he had always worried he'd be a liability to him. Ben said he had always been looking for an opportunity to rekindle the friendship.

"I never lost hope, respect, or love for you," Ben said. "You're always my best friend. My fiancée knows everything about you!"

Aidan still can't really believe this happened. "You're hearing all this come out of the mouth of someone you knew from zero to eighteen, in a voice that is just so slightly changed," he said, "and your memories start to come back and the voice gets more and more familiar until you realize, 'Oh shit, this is my best friend saying these things to me, and he's actually saying them.' And then you hug, you hug it out."

He shook his head. "It was better than I ever could have imagined," he said.

Chapter Twelve

The Thomas Family

As the clock ran down on that fifth game of the season for the San Francisco 49ers—yet another loss, this time at home to the Arizona Cardinals—Martha Thomas sat in a Levi's Stadium box trying to make the most important decision of her life.

She knew her twenty-two-year-old son, Solomon, in his second year as a starting defensive tackle, was in trouble. But she feared that if she told anyone, she could ruin his career.

His only defensive statistic for the entire game was a solo tackle at 4:17 in the first quarter. But it wasn't just that Solly, as he is known, had another lackluster outing on the field. It was what happened, or didn't happen, after he tackled Dennis Johnson at the forty-six-yard line.

"He just got up and walked off the field," Martha told me. "No celebration, no nothing. It looked like he didn't even care that he got a tackle." And when he got back to the sidelines after Arizona was forced to punt, he looked lost. Well-known in San Francisco for his contagious exuberance and animation on and off the field—during his years at Stanford and then as a hometown favorite number three pick in the NFL draft—he now looked dejected, withdrawn, and as small as a muscular, six-foot-three, 280-pound athlete could look.

Solly had suffered a searing tragedy just eight months earlier—Ella, his older sister and closest confidante, had taken her own life at the age of twenty-four. But while his parents seemed to be slowly improving in their bereavement, Solly was actually much worse. He was doing his best to respond to requests that he speak out about suicide prevention in Ella's memory. But he wasn't admitting to anybody that he was suffering from depression and experiencing suicidal ideation himself.

Martha was afraid that she was the only one who realized the danger. But she was also afraid to say anything about it to anyone but Solly. She had been begging him to get help, but he stoically reassured her he was fine.

"*You* get help, Mom," he kept telling her. "*You* get help."

All through the game, she worried. "And I'm really battling in my mind," she said, "do I go to his place of work and tell them that my son needs help? I thought, I can't go—it's his job. He'll never talk to me again. And then I just decided, I don't care if he never talks to me again—as long as he's alive."

When the game was over, Martha hustled down to the special lounge, between Levi's Stadium and the team's practice field, where family members meet their players after the game. Instead of going in, she nervously sought out Austin Moss, the team's young director of player engagement, who she had met a couple times and knew was the team's point person for the league's slowly expanding effort to help players confront mental health and addiction issues. Austin was the person that Martha, and Solly, could undoubtedly go to about mental health.

But everyone knew about the stigma attached to even just admitting you might think you have a problem. During Solomon's rookie year, he was told by his fellow players to never, ever be seen sitting next to the team's sports psychologist—not on the bench, not even at lunch—because people would think he was "crazy." And he didn't need any more prejudice against him. He was already having a statistically challenging second year, which had the media calling into question his $28 million four-year contract. And his family had long dealt with racial friction, because his father was Black and his mother was white.

Martha approached Austin and asked if they could speak privately, away from the family lounge. She looked up at him through her silver bangs—Austin had played football too, at Kentucky, before working his way up in the NFL front office—and she did not pull any punches.

"Someone has to help my son," she told him. "I am not gonna lose both of my kids."

What nobody else knew at the time was that she was also at risk of losing her husband, Chris.

I KNEW OF THE THOMAS FAMILY because they were among a number of families in professional sports who had been active in suicide prevention and talking about the need for mental health care through regional nonprofits—theirs is called The Defensive Line, and it especially focuses on young people of color. It is based in their hometown of Coppell, Texas, a small bedroom community twenty miles outside of Dallas where Solomon played football, and Ella played basketball, for the Coppell Cowboys. But while the family had told isolated parts of their story for good advocacy reasons, as I got to know them through interviews, I realized how important and impactful it could be to bring their whole journey together in one place. Their story shows just how complex and challenging it is for families to handle mental illness and addiction in multiple members simultaneously—even when, in the public eye, they may all seem to be doing great.

Chris and Martha Thomas met in Ohio in the early 1980s, at the small liberal arts school College of Wooster, about forty-five minutes southwest of Akron. Martha had grown up in Northfield, Minnesota, where her father was a United Methodist minister and her mother, a teacher, was active in running community organizations. Martha didn't have much experience with mental illness or addiction growing up: alcohol wasn't allowed in her home, and the only experience she had with mental health was a severely ill woman that her church community helped care for. Her closest experience of mental illness was homesickness when she went away to college. She was a strong student and an athlete, running track in high school and college.

Chris grew up in the small Ohio town of Cambridge and had a more challenging childhood—with more exposure to mental illness, addiction, and abuse. He was raised primarily by his mother, who was a nurse's aide at the local Cambridge State Hospital, which treated patients with psychiatric illnesses and developmental disabilities. While sober herself, she described her family as "drunks," and Chris's enduring image of his maternal grandparents was that "they were always drinking Blatz Beer," a Milwaukee brand.

His father, a gifted semi-pro athlete in basketball, football, and boxing, was "quite absent from our household," he recalled; he traveled around the country and, besides Chris and his two siblings, had children with several other women, "before, during, and after" his marriage to Chris's mom. When his father was home, his parents often fought, and sometimes it got physical. Money was tight. His parents divorced when he was a senior in high school.

Chris described himself as "a survivor of physical, verbal, racial, and sexual abuse." The sexual abuse came from a relative who suffered from mental illness, the physical abuse primarily from his father, who he recalled hitting him, using "whatever he could get his hands on for a beating, whether it was a stick or a belt or, you know, a piece of track from my Hot Wheels set."

While Chris played sports in high school and college—he excelled at track and basketball—his career track was pre-law. He met Martha when he was a junior and she was a freshman, studying history. Their relationship was readily accepted by her parents in Minnesota; Chris was amazed to find out that Martha's father had been involved in the civil rights movement and had once marched with Martin Luther King. Chris's family, on the other hand, was outraged that he was in love with a white woman. So, from the very beginning of their relationship, they experienced the challenges of racial prejudice.

While Chris had planned to go to law school, he was heavily recruited by Procter & Gamble and chose instead to build a career there in sales and management. He began in Columbus, Ohio, and after Martha graduated and they got married in 1985, they moved to Cleveland, where she got a job teaching. They faced prejudice there, even in trying to go to local nightclubs. (They ended up joining a class action suit against one club that wouldn't let them in together.) When Chris was relocated to Cincinnati, they had trouble getting a mortgage because of redlining.

Later the company moved Chris and Martha to Chicago, where they lived in the suburb of Naperville and Martha taught in a Catholic school on the South Side. Their daughter Ella was born there in 1993, nine weeks premature and weighing just three pounds.

"I remember the doctor saying that if she survives, she could be very sick or have severe learning disabilities," Martha said. "But while she didn't really crawl, she rolled—and she was slower to read and later had ADHD—she did fine."

Two years later, Solomon was born. When Solly was two, Procter & Gamble asked Chris to move the family to Sydney, Australia, to oversee their cosmetics and skin care business there. The job was supposed to be for a year, but they ended up staying for five, as Chris was promoted to manage sales and business development for the entire country. So, Ella and Solomon spent their childhood in a unique multicultural society.

Chris rose at Procter & Gamble, in what he described as "a big work-hard, play-hard environment. And I think I played hard a lot." While he had tried to stay away from alcohol while growing up—he saw how it had affected other family members—he had, as a young professional, started drinking socially, primarily Chardonnay and cocktails.

"I started drinking more heavily there," he said. "And I think part of that was that I felt like I didn't really deserve to be where I was at in my career, that I had, like, imposter syndrome."

When the family came back to the United States, he took over Procter & Gamble's Clairol hair color division, based in Stamford, Connecticut. The family lived there for three years, during which Ella and Solly did speech therapy to get rid of their thick Australian accents. Ella was also evaluated for ADHD at All Kinds of Minds, then a well-known neurodevelopmental institute in New York.

During that time, Chris was flying all over the country for work, and felt even more pressure to succeed, "which meant more hiding my lack of self-confidence and my concern about being called out." It also led to more drinking. Chris found himself spending more time in airport lounges, "where I could drink Bloody Marys and Screwdrivers. And then I started to organize my travel schedule so I could be at the airport lounge before I took off, and a lot of times I would try to leave a day before I needed to so I could be sober by the time the meetings started. Eventually, I sometimes drank during the days of meetings, too."

Martha did her best to try to discourage Chris from drinking without confronting him. It didn't work. Finally, Chris got in trouble with Procter & Gamble during a Clairol business trip to Brazil.

"I drank a lot the night before," he told me, "and I got to a meeting like two or three hours late, and then I missed a meeting. And my boss finally just pulled me aside and said, 'Look, this is not good. You're at the point where you might want to think about some other options.' They offered me a position where I could rehabilitate my image. But it meant going back to live in Cincinnati, which we didn't want to do."

Chris didn't tell anyone, including Martha, any of this, because he was embarrassed and scared. Instead, he quietly left Procter & Gamble after more than twenty years with the company. He found a position with Alberto-Culver—global head of sales for their ethnic hair care business—which he also could spin as a better opportunity. Nobody needed to know the role that alcohol use had played in his career.

The new job was based in Dallas, where he and Martha and the kids moved in 2005. Ella was twelve, Solly was ten, but they were three years apart in school. Chris continued to travel all over for work, but the kids spent the rest of their formative years there, in the suburb of Coppell, where they started in the same public school system where Martha eventually got a job teaching. She began as a regular sub, but eventually not only taught middle school but also coached a variety of sports—and became so active that she even drove the school bus to first-thing-in-the-morning practices. As a result, she often left for school before her kids.

Ella and Solly both were attractive, athletic, and perhaps a little more emotional than they appeared. Solly saw his older sister as much tougher than he was, even though he started growing bigger than her by the third grade. "She could still get the best of me when we would wrestle and roughhouse," he recalled. "There's a saying that you have to be a little mean to play football. I'm kind of a soft-spoken guy, so at Stanford, my D-line coach asked where I got my meanness. I told him that, honestly, I got beat up too many times by my sister." Any youthful friction between them ended after the brother of Ella's best friend died of a drug overdose when Ella was in eleventh grade and Solly in eighth. After that, they made a pact to be "the best we can be to each other."

Ella had some learning issues and some childhood behaviors she didn't outgrow: at home, while she stopped sucking her thumb, she was still comforted by a stuffed animal from her childhood—originally a lamb named Lamby, which was lost on a family trip and replaced by a dog, Puppers. She needed extra help in school, and soon after moving to Texas, reluctantly started taking medication for her ADHD. Martha tried to get her registered for disability assistance but was frustrated to learn that, in Texas, she couldn't.

"She had the diagnosis, but never did badly enough in school, if that makes any sense, to qualify," Martha said, fuming. "When we lived in Connecticut, she would have received assistance with that diagnosis. In Texas, nothing."

But her learning differences never stopped her from being popular at school and a protective older sister. "Ella was very easy," Martha said. "She could always get along. She got along with a *tree*, you know?" She was also a good athlete, especially strong in basketball. She was also involved in helping people experiencing homelessness, especially after going on a church mission to Chicago. "She often took any money we gave her for anything and gave it to the disadvantaged," Martha said.

Solomon played sports, but he was equally interested in theater. "Everything is competitive here in Texas," Martha joked, "so he had to audition for theater class, and they said he could do it alongside football. So, as a freshman in high school, he was sometimes at school from 6:00 A.M. to 10:00 P.M. so he could do both. I would bring him breakfast and dinner at school."

By then, however, Solly had grown dramatically out of his chunkiness and the braces on his teeth, and it was clear he had the size and advancing skill to focus on athletics. Theater took a backseat, and by the time he was a sophomore at Coppell High School, scouts started paying attention to him. He went from watching *Friday Night Lights* to living it.

Chris's job at Alberto-Culver lasted only two years. He was then hired by Frito-Lay to oversee custom sales for Walmart, which was based in Arkansas. He bought a condo in Fayetteville and commuted for two years. When the company moved him back near Dallas, the family decided to keep the condo. It was part of the reason why Ella decided to attend the University of Arkansas, which was in the same town. Fayetteville was nearly five hours away from Coppell, but it was an easy place for her parents to stay when they visited her. Some smaller schools had looked at Ella as a possible college basketball recruit, but she said she was done with sports.

Martha was initially optimistic about the move for Ella. It was a fresh start, and under Arkansas rules, Ella would qualify for special help and extra time on tests because of her ADHD. Unfortunately, when the two of them went together to get Ella registered at the Equal Opportunity Compliance office on the Fayetteville campus, they found the people there dismissive.

"Ella comes in," Martha remembered, "and she's beautiful and looks very put together, and they were really rude to her. I'm sure there were other reasons. One, she's a Black girl coming in with a white mother. And she doesn't have a visible enough handicap. Like, there were people there in wheelchairs."

Martha watched the whole thing unfold, and was not surprised when Ella just said "Screw it." But she understood that something she had hoped would give Ella a better chance in college had instead turned into a very early and meaningful setback.

ELLA STRUGGLED THROUGH much of her freshman year at Arkansas. Besides her anxiety and depression, she had developed gastrointestinal problems, which ran in Martha's family. But Ella came home for the summer, regrouped, and returned with more confidence to start her sophomore year. This was partially fueled by the growing excitement in the family about Solomon, whose star was rising among college scouts all over the country. He looked like he could even be NFL bound.

But that fall, Solly and Ella both experienced stunning tragedies. One was covered in newspapers all over Texas. The other wasn't discovered by the family until years later, after it had already created so much complicated trauma.

One of Solly's best friends on the Coppell team was senior wide receiver Jacob Logan. The two of them were team leaders, and also had something else in common: both had Black fathers and white mothers. To directly confront any small-town Texas prejudice, they proudly referred to themselves as "hybrids," which became popular enough around school that during one game, fans in the stands took off their shirts to reveal the words "hybrid" on their chests and "nation" on their backs. (*Dallas* magazine said the two "made being biracial cool.")

One Sunday in mid-October, several of Solly's friends from the team were outside of town at Possum Kingdom Lake, boating and swimming. Solly couldn't join them because he had to catch up on homework; he had spent the day before at the annual Texas–Oklahoma game being recruited by both team's coaches.

On the south end of the lake, there were legendary, dramatic cliffs that people dove from even though it was risky. Jacob and another friend from the team had never done it before. As the two climbed up the sixty-foot cliff, Jacob reportedly told his friend, "If God wants to take me, he'll take me." The friend jumped first, and successfully swam back to the boat. Then Jacob jumped, landing feet first. He surfaced for a moment, to everyone's relief, but then he went under again. And he never came back up.

Two days later, as divers were still searching for his body, the school was rocked again as one of the young men who carried flags during football games and did push-ups after every touchdown took his own life. On Thursday, Jacob's body was finally found. And then Friday night, the team had to play. Before the game, Solly was the one who led Jacob's sister, Jordan—wearing her late brother's #21 jersey—out onto the field. He was able to hold it together for himself and his team—which won the game and went on to finish the season undefeated—because he had the support of his family, as well as the first mental health professional he ever met.

"There was a school counselor the district sent in," Solly told me.

"I still remember his name, Mr. Hagen. He was a very soothing man. I really appreciated his time and he made a big impact on me. I was spending a lot of time and energy being there for other people and making sure everyone was loving on Jacob's family. But I wasn't really looking at myself. And I remember Mr. Hagen always asking me questions and taking me in during class and seeing how I was doing."

Even the media took note at how emotional Solly was for a top national football recruit. He was described on ESPN.com as a "defensive end with the game-day look of someone you want to steer clear of but who has a heart twice the size of Texas."

WHILE SOLOMON WAS getting the support he needed to process his friend's death, neither he nor his parents knew just how much help his sister Ella desperately needed, and didn't know how to ask for, during this same time.

One weekend during that same fall of 2012—nobody ever learned exactly which one—Ella Thomas was gang-raped at a fraternity party on the University of Arkansas campus. Her family never learned too many details; Ella waited two years to share with her parents what had happened to her, and then she asked them to keep it a secret. She waited even longer to tell Solly what had happened.

The only details they ever learned about the horrifying incident were that Ella had been drinking, so when she quietly explored trying to report the incident, she was told she couldn't. "She said she was told that in Arkansas," Martha said, "the laws were that if you had gone to a party and there were witnesses to you drinking or using, if something went wrong, they were not liable. I don't know for sure if that's what she was told, but she said that was why she didn't pursue it."

Solomon's understanding was "she tried to tell people at the school, but they didn't do anything. In the end, she must have felt like it was her fault."

But, at the time, all they knew was that when Ella came home to Texas from Arkansas for Thanksgiving break in 2012, she seemed like a different person.

"It almost seemed like her light was being snuffed out," Martha recalled. "She just didn't seem like herself. She always had such great energy, such great, well, *light.* And suddenly it was gone. She was more angry. We noticed right away, of course. And I remember asking her lots of times, over that break and the next several months, what was going on with her, what was wrong.

"And, she just said, 'Nothing, there's nothing wrong.'"

Ella returned to school for her spring semester, but her grades plummeted. Martha tried to help her arrange appointments with counselors on campus, but she wouldn't go. Eventually, Solomon would later recall, "She dropped out and didn't tell us why. Then, almost back to back, a close college friend of hers died and two other acquaintances died in a boat crash. Her depression got worse and worse."

Because the family still had the condo in Fayetteville, Ella had remained there as she faltered in school. She got a job there and would make the drive home to Coppell often—for holidays, even for Solly's football games.

During his senior year, Solly was the subject of major national recruiting attention. He had seventy-eight tackles that year, and twelve and a half sacks. It was exciting, and distracting enough that Ella's new challenges, which they didn't realize included intense, untreated PTSD, became her new normal.

The same was true of Chris's ongoing struggle with drinking, which had led him to change jobs twice since Solly was in high school. "This was the beginning of me starting to drink at work, that kind of stuff," he recalled. "I was just taking these easy jobs to make some money and get some benefits."

His most recent job was with a company based in St. Cloud, Minnesota. In the fall of 2013, during the height of Solly's recruitment, Chris drank at the airport in Dallas before flying to Minnesota, drank after landing at a bar there, and then went to a Burger King where he was reportedly slurring his words so much when he ordered that they called the police while he was waiting for his food. He was pulled over after leaving the parking lot. He spent six hours in jail, got out on bail, and never told his family about it. He was able to plead to charges and nearly made the whole thing go away without Martha finding out. The first she ever heard of it was over a year later, when a letter about his rehabilitation training was sent to their house in Texas instead of his work, and she opened it.

By the winter, Solly had narrowed his college choices down to two schools in California—Stanford and UCLA. But he was also still considering the University of Arkansas. "I actually almost went to Arkansas instead of Stanford," he would later write in an open letter to his late sister, "because that's where my big sister was. I couldn't have cared less what the football team was like there. I wanted to go there because I knew . . . as much as I needed you, you needed me, too. I don't regret going to Stanford . . . and you never resented me or made me feel bad for not joining you at Arkansas. But . . . it's hard not to think that maybe things could've been different had I made that choice—if I had been around you more . . . when you were really struggling."

SOLLY DIDN'T PLAY his freshman year at Stanford; as is often the case for top prospects, he was redshirted to preserve four more years of eligibility as he developed. During his redshirt year, he took a management course with a unique classmate: John Lynch, a former Stanford and NFL player, then doing color commentary for the NFL on Fox, who had decided to finish his college degree. The two got to know each other while working on a group project together.

In his sophomore year, Solly played all fourteen games, amassing thirty-nine tackles for the year, capped off with a fumble recovery for a touchdown in the PAC-12 Championship against USC. In the post-season, he had four tackles, including a sack, in the Rose Bowl.

His junior year, in the fall of 2016, went even better on the field, with sixty-two tackles. But he spent much of that season under pressure trying to decide whether to quit school and go professional. He started working with a sports psychologist that the team offered to players.

"I started getting a little stressed about making the decision whether I should leave school or not," he recalled. "I was playing really well and having a good year. Then we started losing a couple games. I really wanted to win, and I didn't know what to do about the decision. We started off talking about that."

But it wasn't very long before the conversations with the psychologist began focusing on his sister, Ella, "and how worried I was about her. Ella had been calling, telling me that she was struggling in her relationships, struggling in Arkansas, it was tough. She was out of school, still hoping to go back. She was bartending there, just to make money." Ella had told Solly that she always felt like she was only one step ahead of her depression and anxiety, and it kept catching up to her. She had trouble sleeping.

By this time, Solly and his parents knew about Ella's rape in college and were coming to understand its impact on her. She had spent years trying to get it out of her mind rather than seeking treatment.

While they don't remember the exact date—except that it was sometime during the 2014–2015 school year—both Martha and Chris have vivid memories of Ella, home from Arkansas, finally telling them the truth.

They remember being sound asleep and Ella coming into their bedroom and waking them up. "She said, 'I need to tell you guys something. I need to tell you what happened,'" Martha recalled. "She didn't go into any details, just that she had been gang-raped at a fraternity party two years before, and she wasn't doing well. I remember the three of us just sitting on the bedroom floor, hugging each other and crying."

Not only did they feel incredible pain for their daughter and sympathy for her trauma, but there was also an odd sense of relief.

For so long, Martha had been asking herself what had happened to Ella that had so changed her life in college. Ella had reassured her so many times that nothing had happened that she had almost come to believe it. Now she finally knew.

"Oh my god," Martha kept saying to herself. "*That's* what happened! *That's* what happened."

Both Martha and Chris recall discussing the revelation privately with Solomon not long after. Solomon doesn't remember it that way, saying he heard about it directly from Ella, but several months later. Either way, by the fall of 2016, while Ella was struggling in Arkansas, Solly was in California feeling nervous about his future and scared for his sister.

One day while he was in a meeting, Ella texted him a photo showing where she had cut herself on the arm and explaining, he recalled, "she was going through a lot of pain, but it was going to make her stronger." He immediately ran out of the meeting room to call her. "We talked on the phone for thirty minutes, during which she was crying. I was just trying to calm her down, telling her things were going to be okay." It was the first time she had ever reached out to him for help.

"The sports psychologist gave me a couple of numbers in Arkansas that I could get to Ella for, like, a domestic violence hotline or something like that," he recalled. "But I didn't want to risk my trust with Ella and tell my parents I was worried. I didn't have a lot of money at the time, but I had some left from my college stipend, and I found a way to send it to her, so she could do whatever she needed—whether she needed some independence or some help."

Did you frame this to her that she could use it to get therapy, to get mental health care, I wondered.

"No, I didn't really understand what therapy was at that point," he said. "What I was doing with the sports psychologist, that was sports psychology, not therapy." It was more of a supportive pep talk to improve performance on the field. Therapy was something different.

"When I thought about therapy," Solly said, "I thought, like, *what* is wrong with you?" If going to a sports psychologist meant there was something wrong with him, he probably wouldn't have gone.

SOLLY DECLARED HIS ELIGIBILITY for the draft after the 2016 season, which ended triumphantly with Stanford holding on to beat North Carolina in the Sun Bowl. Solly had seven tackles, including a dramatic third-down sack with less than three minutes to play. He didn't return to school for the spring 2017 semester, and the family got entirely caught up in his football career drama. In an unorthodox move, the 49ers hired John Lynch—the veteran NFL player turned announcer who had been in Solly's freshman management class—as its new general manager, the head of the team. And the Thomases were all together in Philadelphia in April for the NFL draft, during which Lynch surprised a lot of people by selecting Solly as the third pick of the first round.

Solly stood to earn a rookie contract of over $28 million for four years, guaranteed, including a signing bonus of over $18 million, but the negotiations dragged on longer than expected, well into the summer.

For months, Solly shuttled between California—where he crashed at a friend's house—and Texas. During this same period, Martha remembered Ella being thrilled for her brother but struggling even more personally. In the early summer, she left Arkansas for good—the family had sold their condo there and she had been renting while working as a bartender. She moved back home with her dog, Mickey, a pit bull/boxer mix, into her old bedroom.

When Solly was home, he and Ella did what they always had done. They drove together on long Texas roads with the music blaring in the car. They played hoops. They sat together on a family room couch—Ella clutching her stuffed animal Puppers—while they watched their favorite movies: *Step Brothers, The Hangover, Bad Boys 2.*

Sometimes Ella seemed like she was doing better, but that feeling never seemed to last long. She had a good job as a bartender. She did weight training to get in better shape. She could look beautiful and composed when she absolutely needed to. But now that she was living at home for the first time since high school, it was clear that her day-to-day life was even more of a struggle than her family had realized.

Eventually, Solly's contract negotiation ended. He reported for training camp in the late summer and began his rookie season in the NFL. At the same time, his family settled in—Chris, Martha, and Ella living under the same roof for the first time in years.

On weekends they often flew to his games. The rest of the time, they adjusted to the new normal of Ella being at home, Martha still teaching and coaching during most waking hours, and Chris often being on the road for work. When Chris was home, it was clear his drinking was getting worse. Ella's mental health was also getting worse. But as a veteran bartender, she also knew better than the rest of the family what alcoholism looked like. So, she was the one who confronted Chris about his drinking, which had the added benefit of distracting some of the attention from her own depression and anxiety.

Solomon was worrying about his sister. "The changes in her behavior during my rookie year were definitely more alarming," he recalled. "She would tell stories that didn't add up. Sometimes I would get mad and say, 'Look, I don't know if you're lying to mask your emotions, but it's confusing for me.' I was trying to be her biggest supporter, but at the same time, I was thinking, 'What's going on here?'"

One thing she kept telling him was "I just can't be happy."

He tried to talk her out of this. "What do you mean you can't be happy?" he would say. "Yes, you can be happy."

And she would say, "No, I can't, it's just not there for me."

"I just didn't understand what she meant," he told me. "I just didn't understand the pressure of it, the anxiety of it, didn't understand the chemistry of it, the science of it, that it's a real thing in the makeup of your brain that is not allowing you to be happy. I just thought you could control your happiness, and find ways to be perceptive and have a different perspective, and find happiness. So, when she said that, I thought she was *choosing* not to be happy."

Solly's rookie season was also challenging, apart from his concern about Ella. He was playing a different defensive position than he had in high school and college on a 49ers team that was clearly rebuilding. They had a first-time general manager who hired a first-time coach, and they opened the season with nine straight losses. It wasn't until mid-November that they won their first game.

Over Thanksgiving, the family came to visit because the team had a Sunday home game. Ella stayed at the house Solomon was renting, and since she didn't like the bed in the guest room, she slept in the living room.

"I was going to work out very early one morning," he recalled, "and she was sleeping on the couch. I knew she had PTSD, she had told me about the rape, but I'm not sure I really knew what that meant. And then all of a sudden, at five in the morning she looked like she was wide-awake having a panic attack, but she was dead asleep. She was, like, having spastic movements, shaking from side to side. And I was yelling 'Ella, Ella, wake up!' but she was legit asleep. And that's when I started thinking, 'Oh shit, Ella is really messed up right now.' She was definitely raped, she is definitely struggling, she definitely can't be happy right now, something is definitely wrong with her."

The team lost that Sunday, but won the next two. Chris, Martha, and Ella came to San Francisco for Christmas because Solly had a Christmas Eve Day home game against the Jaguars. They won, and Solly did well, especially in the second quarter when he made a tackle on first down, and then sacked the quarterback on second down. After the game, Ella, Martha, and Solly attended the team's gala Christmas party. They were all pleased to see how happy and comfortable Ella was among the players and their families.

"It was great," Martha recalled. "Ella really turned heads. There was a dinner and drinking and lots of beautiful people, and she just flitted around and had a great time. She loved it. She fit in. There were hundreds of people, like everyone that worked for the Niners and their families. I remember watching her, and watching people watch her. She was great at a party, great around people."

It was being by herself that was so challenging.

Solomon moved back to Texas after the season, hoping it would help to be closer to Ella. He also had work to do in the off-season: considered to be a little small by NFL standards, he had bulked up from 272 to 280 for his rookie year, but the consensus was that he needed to put on even more muscle to reach his full potential.

By the time Solly returned home, just a week or two after Christmas, Ella was much worse. She had a therapist, but it was unclear if she was actually going to her appointments. She was taking the anti-anxiety medicine alprazolam (Xanax), but Solomon wasn't sure if these were the pills she previously had been prescribed, or if she was buying them from friends at the bar where she worked—and possibly had become addicted to them. She had a boyfriend that her family didn't like very much. And she seemed not only depressed and anxious as she had been, but angry in a way that seemed new.

"Just before I got home, she was reaching out all the time, 'Solly I need you at home, I can't wait to see you, I need to hug you,'" he recalled. "Then I got home and she wasn't around that much. Or, maybe she was there, but not really there. She was saying she couldn't live at home anymore, it was hard being around Mom and Dad. She said she felt suffocated." There was also an issue that he had given her some money for Christmas so she could buy a new car, but then found out from his mom that Ella was spending it elsewhere.

While things were, as Solly recalled, "definitely a little more weird," none of them had any idea of the possible danger. It just wasn't anything they could imagine.

As Chris told me when I first met him, "I honestly didn't know Black people died by suicide."

ON THE EVENING of January 22, 2018, Ella went to stay at her boyfriend's apartment. Martha urged her to just stay home. "I asked her not to leave the house that night," she recalled. "I said, 'Don't go over there. Just stay here. You know, stay home.' And she said, 'You know what, Mom, my work clothes are over there, he's got the late shift so he won't get home till 3:00 or 4:00 in the morning. I really won't have to see him. And I'll be leaving fairly early.'"

First thing in the morning, Ella did text Martha, who was already at school by 7:00 A.M., sitting at her middle school classroom desk reading from her phone.

"She wrote, 'I love you, never forget how much I love you,'" Martha recalled. "This was not necessarily unusual, she often texted that to me, and I would text the same thing back to her." She texted back that she loved Ella, too, and asked what she was doing up so early. She didn't answer, but Martha had to start teaching.

When she was able to look at her phone again between morning classes, Martha noticed something strange. Ella was supposed to have left for work, to be there at 11:00 A.M., but the location indicator on her phone said she was still at her boyfriend's apartment. And she was no longer texting Martha back.

After more unanswered texts, Martha found a phone number for the boyfriend, who she assumed had come back late at night and was sleeping out on the couch. When Martha finally reached him by text at 1:42 P.M., he wrote back, "She's still here. She has locked herself in my room because we got into it last night." Martha urged him to check on her.

"I didn't hear from him for a while," she recalled, "and then he called me and said, 'You should get over here. She shot herself.'"

She ran to the principal's office and he drove her to the apartment. By the time they arrived, the police were there. They had broken the bedroom door down. And Ella was already gone. The police told her Ella had not died right away after shooting herself in the chest. She was reportedly found in the exact position Martha would have expected—holding Puppers. Martha was taken to a police car. Her principal called Chris, who was out of town on business. Chris called Solly.

Because it was the boyfriend's gun and the situation was unusual, Ella's death was investigated as a possible homicide or suicide. Martha didn't want it to be suicide, but she wasn't sure what to think between her own emotions and the mixed signals from the police. Eventually, they were able to break the password of Ella's cell phone. When they did, they found a text she sent to a friend saying she couldn't take it anymore and evidence that she had watched a video on YouTube about how to shoot the type of gun her boyfriend had. Investigators ultimately ruled that Ella had taken her own life, but called it an "impulsive and aggravated suicide."

BESIDES THE HUGE funeral for Ella in Coppell—attended by many 49ers players, coaches, and executives—Solly, Martha, and Chris withdrew from their public lives for months. Martha took a leave of absence from teaching, Chris stopped working, Solly remained in Texas and did nothing but work out. Martha was the first to try to return to her life—after six weeks she started teaching again. But she knew immediately she had gone back too soon.

"I was still crying, and not knowing I was crying," she recalled. "I remember the kids telling me, the first day I was back, 'Mrs. Thomas, your cheeks are wet.' I was, like, 'Wow, I didn't know.'"

Solly posted on Instagram about Ella right away: "My sweet, sweet Ella you will forever be missed. As this is not a goodbye. You are forever by my side. Forever. Thank you for everything, Ella. We ride together, we die together, Bad Boys for life." But it was nearly four months before the family started speaking about Ella's death and life, with the encouragement of the American Foundation for Suicide Prevention, to highlight the family's upcoming participation in an AFSP "Out of the Darkness Overnight Walk" in Dallas. Solly wrote something for the organization's web page, and he spoke to the press in San Francisco and in Dallas.

He was honest from the beginning that he was having a very hard time when he was alone, his brain flooded with "what ifs" and "how could we not have knowns" and his heart aching from not being able to text or call or hug Ella just one more time. But he was also very good at sharing these feelings, exactly what was needed for suicide prevention advocacy.

Solly followed in the footsteps of other athletes who were speaking up about family members lost to suicide (as well as sports colleagues lost to suicide, sometimes, presumably, because of brain damage from concussions). But he was also inspired by athletes like basketball star Kevin Love who talked openly about their own mental health struggles and the challenges of treatment.

He and his family quickly embraced the concept of extended, complex grief and the support available for those experiencing it. They were less ready to embrace the possibility that they were struggling with more than just grief over losing Ella. Chris had an alcohol use disorder that had been getting worse even before Ella had taken her life. And while Solly was an inspiring public figure who had handled public tragedy since high school, he was perhaps a little too good at delivering the right advocacy message and seeming mentally healthy without always acknowledging his own struggles.

The first hint the team had of a disconnect between Solly's public persona as a growing advocate and his own inner turmoil came at the very beginning of training camp in late July. Austin Moss, a former college football player himself, had just recently been hired as director of player engagement by the team, after working several years at the NFL main offices helping develop the league's response to mental health and addiction issues. He also suddenly had a French bulldog in his office—which he had agreed to dog-sit for a few weeks for a fellow employee.

Everyone on the team was watching Solly as he reconnected, and many were concerned that he didn't seem himself. Austin was buoyed that as soon as Solomon saw the dog in his office, he wanted to come play with it whenever he had free time.

"It was the one moment that I got to see him express any type of joy or happiness," Austin told me. "It was just like he was so much like himself again in that moment." The dog reminded Solly of Ella's dog, Mickey.

After visiting the dog every day for a few days, Solly made a surprising proposal. "He came to me," Austin recalled, "and asked 'Would you be willing to see if we can get the dog here full time?' He said it could be an 'emotional support animal' because it was really helping him a lot."

At first Austin was hesitant. He was new to the team, and this would be an unusual request to run up the chain of command. And a dog in the locker room could be a distraction. He also couldn't keep the bulldog he was dog-sitting for a friend; he would actually have to go buy another bulldog, and keep it himself, just so Solly could have the emotional support. But the team approved—it didn't hurt that Solly and the GM were friends—and Austin and Solly went and bought a French bulldog from the same breeder as the one he had been dog-sitting. They named her Zoe, and she was in Austin's office whenever Solly, or any player, wanted to play with her.

It wasn't long before Solly needed the extra support. During the first quarter of the first preseason game against the Cowboys, he was knocked unconscious by hitting the ground hard after a third-down stop.

To make things worse, while this was happening, Chris was up in one of the stadium boxes with friends and had already had so much to drink that he didn't even notice his son was injured.

"This is not one of my proud moments of being a parent," he told me, "but Martha had to call me from Dallas—it was a Thursday game and she couldn't come because she had to coach—and tell me Solly was hurt on the field. I was drunk and did not know he was hurting."

Martha was incensed. "Solly was out cold, and they showed it a little on TV and then they cut the camera away," she remembered. "I wanted to know what was happening, and that's when I realized Chris wasn't coherent. And this wasn't the first time this had happened. It was an ongoing problem. Solly later talked to Chris, and said if he was going to continue to be drunk at games, he wasn't going to be welcome. We actually talked about Chris agreeing that he would have a one-drink limit for each half. This had been a problem before, but it got much worse after Ella's death."

Fortunately, Solly regained consciousness and left the field under his own power. But he underwent the NFL concussion protocol for the next few weeks.

"It sucked," he recalled. "I had headaches all the time. And you have to be in darkness a lot. I was already depressed before the concussion. Those two weeks in darkness didn't help." He was able to return to play the last game of the preseason.

As soon as the season started, it was clear Solly still wasn't himself on the field. He lacked his well-appreciated high energy both on the field and on the sidelines. The first game he had no solo tackles and just one assist, and the next three games he had just one or two solo tackles. But while there wasn't much to say about his playing, he was suddenly very much in demand to do in-depth interviews about Ella's suicide and sports mental health. Martha and Chris were pretty sure he wasn't ready to do this yet, and some of the 49ers staff were also unsure. But Solly was committed to doing what he perceived to be the right thing for Ella.

"We were worried," Martha admitted. Solly did two big interviews with ESPN, one for its magazine, which ran as an "as told to" on September 18, and another on camera, which was being prepared to run during ESPN's *Countdown* show before *Monday Night Football* on October 15, when the 49ers would play the Packers. "They asked us if we would be part of the interview," Martha told me. "Even though I didn't want to do it, and I didn't think Solly should do it, I wasn't going to let him do it himself." As they watched him being filmed, they saw how many times Solly ducked his head, and started rubbing it and said he had to stop and walk off camera. To her it looked less like an effective call for advocacy and more like a cry for help.

All of which led Martha to pull Austin Moss aside after the October 7 Cardinals game and urge him to let somebody with the team—preferably GM John Lynch—know that she felt Solly would never get the help he needed unless the 49ers told him it was not only okay but something they really thought he should do.

Moss knew Martha for an ironic reason—only weeks before, the team had brought her and Chris in to be on a panel for the rookie family symposium to share with players' parents how they had coped during their son's first year in the NFL. Now she was admitting how worried she was about Solly.

Moss immediately reached out to the GM's office for permission to arrange a meeting between Solly and an outside psychologist the team had a relationship with. GM John Lynch made the first outreach himself.

"We were in the cafeteria," Solly recalled, "and my general manager came up to me and said, 'Solly, we know you're struggling. If you need any help, we have your back.' I went home that night and looked at myself in the mirror. And I was, like, 'Dude, I've been thinking about killing myself and not being here for about two or three months now. I think I need help.'"

By October 9, Austin had an email confirming Solly's first appointment. When the ESPN *Monday Night Football Countdown* interview ran several days later, Solly was already getting therapy, and admitting to the psychologist things he hadn't told anyone else.

He was profoundly depressed. He could fake it when he was around other people, but as soon as he was by himself, he was lost. He was thinking more and more often about, as he explained it to me, "not being here anymore. I just didn't see any light in the future. I've lost people before. When Jacob died I was, of course, very sad and I missed him and felt grief. But I didn't think there was anything wrong with me. Now I did. I felt like I was losing my life, almost.

"I would go home after practice, and I had two roommates at the time in Menlo Park, and we would come home and joke around and have a good time. But then when I went to my room, everything was dark. I was thinking, 'I don't like it here, I don't want to be here.' I was thinking about ending my life, dying by suicide. And I was even landing on methods in my head for not being here. And these just became my thoughts. Thinking about dying became a normal, day-to-day thing. I knew it wasn't normal, but it was feeling more and more normal. And I just really didn't know how to handle it."

Solly had four sessions with the psychologist, as the team had suggested, and then decided he wanted to continue working with her. Progress was slow but steady. He tried traditional talk therapy. He was encouraged to journal about his feelings and his memories, which especially appealed to him because of all the alone time during the season. Solly told me he did not try any medication, nor was it suggested he should. Later that year, his father started taking the antidepressant escitalopram (Lexapro).

The season ended up being a disaster for the 49ers—who finished 4 and 12, second-worst in the NFL—and a setback for Solly, who played two more games than he had as a rookie, but had ten fewer tackles for the season. Still, he committed to his mental health treatment in the same way he committed to any other medical care or self-improvement. He took it seriously, and even though he was not well, he was still willing to counsel other players who were going through problems themselves or in their families. He also kept seeing the psychologist he had met through the team, hiring her separately—first to work with him directly, and then to see his parents, and then the three of them together.

"Guys are definitely wary of talking about depression and anxiety and panic attacks and PTSD with the team sports psychologist," Solly noted. "Today, when I talk to athletes about mental health, I always recommend they get help from a professional not associated with the team. You're just always less likely to communicate in a vulnerable, raw way if the team is providing the therapy."

He became a strong advocate for athletes to get the mental health care they need, and admits "it's still hard for guys to speak up about this in my profession." It is easier for some players to discuss getting therapy than taking medication, "but to me it's the same thing. Look, from an NFL perspective, it's hard enough just to say you're going through something. I definitely have had teammates who were on antianxiety medication." He is also mindful of the difference between feeling depressed and sad, and having diagnosable depressive illness. "I have been pretty depressed," he said, "but I've never been diagnosed with depression or anything like that. I am, generally, more emotional, but I can't go around and say I've been diagnosed with depression."

The Thomases worked with the psychologist for the better part of a year. They continued all the way through the 2019 season, which was a breakthrough for the 49ers, who improved from 4–12 to a record of 13–3, and went to the Super Bowl. But statistically, it was Solly's least productive year. He played in the Super Bowl but did not record a tackle. But he did his best to maintain his optimism, keep with his mental health regimen, and continue doing advocacy in Ella's memory.

It turned out to be lucky that the family was still in therapy together in March 2020, when Chris was arrested for driving under the influence in California. He had been staying at Solly's house on a business trip while Solly was back in Texas training. He went out to buy another bottle of wine and was pulled over by the police just as he returned to Solly's house.

"I got picked up for DUI and I ended up in the county jail, with real criminals, for two days because I didn't want to call Martha and Solly and tell them what happened," he told me. "I thought I would just be able to talk my way out of it—going to court, getting released on my own recognizance—but I wasn't able to. After two days I finally had to just call and say 'Look, I'm in jail and here's why.'"

Martha and Solly actually already knew where Chris was. When he stopped returning phone calls and texts, they started frantically looking for him and discovered what had happened.

They had him bailed out, but Martha told him not to come home. She had talked about this with the therapist and decided that if he didn't get serious residential care for his alcoholism, she was done. She had found him a place called La Hacienda in Texas Hill Country near Austin. If he agreed, she would arrange for him to go directly there—he couldn't come home first. And if he refused to go for treatment, he couldn't come home at all.

"I'm arranging for all this before school starts in the morning, and in between classes, because otherwise people don't answer their phones at the end of the day" she recalled. "So the students are saying, 'I wonder what's going on with Mrs. Thomas.'" She arranged for Chris to fly back, and when he got to the airport, it was nearly deserted. It turned out he was flying on one of the first days the COVID pandemic hit with full force. The facility had him picked up at the San Antonio airport, and he went straight there. Nobody was allowed to visit.

And then Martha and Solly just waited.

"One day Solomon said to me, 'Why are you so sad?'" she recalled. "And I was thinking, well, let's see. If I'm happy even twenty percent of the time right now, I think that's pretty good. Our daughter died. Solly was still at the stage where he was trying to stuff things away. And my husband is in treatment, and I don't know if he's going to choose me or alcohol."

Chris was at La Hacienda for five weeks. He recalled it took only three or four days there, facing the prospect of not returning to his family, to realize "this is not the life I want to live." He learned about his alcoholism. He explored his abuse as a boy and other adverse childhood experiences. He started taking naltrexone (Vivitrol), in pill form to control his urges to drink in addition to his antidepressant. He embraced the twelve steps. Because of COVID, there was no opportunity for Martha and Solly to be part of family meetings or therapy.

"I really didn't know if treatment was going to work for him," Martha recalled. "And, at least so far, it has."

I wondered what she did with twenty years of pent-up frustration after Chris got his treatment and she wasn't included.

"Well, I mean, it's a lot to deal with," she said. "There's a lot of . . . *aftermath*."

Chris came home from residential treatment and shifted into an intensive outpatient program at Grace Counseling, an addiction treatment facility nearby, where he went three times a week, for three hours at a time. He also went to twelve-step meetings: he was supposed to do ninety meetings in ninety days, but did more than one meeting many days. He continued taking naltrexone and escitalopram (as he does to this day).

If all this pressure wasn't enough, during this time, the 49ers announced they would not be picking up the optional fifth year of Solly's contract. So, he would likely be a free agent. He trained to be ready for a year when he would have to impress his next team, but just forty-nine snaps into his fall 2020 season, he tore up his left knee and was done for the year: torn ACL, lateral meniscus, and medial patellofemoral ligament. Surgery and six grueling months of rehab.

He was picked up in March 2021 by the Raiders, who had been in Oakland during his college and early pro career before moving to Las Vegas and had taken a liking to him. He had had disappointing seasons, but his work ethic and his unique openness about mental health and suicide prevention made the Raiders feel he could still fulfill his promise.

Solly moved to Las Vegas, where the first thing he did was find a new therapist. Then in late May 2021, he and his parents started their own nonprofit, The Defensive Line, after years of doing appearances for other groups, especially AFSP and the NFL. The organization's mission was simple: "to help build a world in which no young person of color dies by suicide" through advocacy, programs, and fundraising. It was initially run by their niece, but within a year Martha gave up teaching to work for the foundation full-time, and Chris followed soon after.

Solly had one of his best seasons ever for the Raiders in 2021 and was then signed by the New York Jets. So then he had to find yet another mental health professional.

"What I love about Solly is that he's not afraid to go find a therapist," Martha said. "He had a good therapist in Nevada, but then he moves to New Jersey, and he knows right away he has to do this. And it's just like any doctor, you have to go and try them out. You don't like this guy, you find someone else. He does it for himself, and he helps a lot of fellow players do it, too. He's really good at it. Because he has to be."

AT THE END of our time together, I spoke to Martha and Chris one last time—Solly couldn't join because he had a game coming up in two days. They noted that while it had been more than five years since Ella's death, their son's life and his playing were more together, but his grief and depression—two different things—could still be overwhelming.

They talked about a recent family trip to Vietnam that they had taken during the past off season. During their first jet-lagged night in Hanoi, Martha got a text from Solly after three in the morning—sent from his hotel room just down the hall.

"Mom," he wrote, "what are you doing?"

She went down to his hotel room, and he was very upset. He said that the trip felt so much like the kind of adventure that he and Ella had gone on with Martha and Chris when they were kids. He had also been focusing a lot on Ella's thirtieth birthday, which was just a few weeks away, and how much he missed her. He was thinking about the times that they hadn't had—and would never have.

"He was, like, 'What are we doing here?'" she recalled. "He said, 'We're not supposed to be doing this without Ella.' To him, to be on this trip without her felt like we were cheating on her in some way."

I asked what she meant by "cheating."

"That we are living life without Ella," Martha continued. "Like we live this incredible life, going to Solomon's games and meeting cool people and seeing things all over the country because our son plays in the NFL. But Solomon does this as part of his job, and we do it because we're his parents. But it still doesn't feel right to do it, and enjoy it, without Ella."

Martha remembered sitting there in Solly's hotel room, and saying to him, "You do all this public grieving, but you've got to take care of the private stuff. It's not the same. You know, it's not the same."

Chris was nodding as Martha continued: "You can talk about things publicly. But the stuff you do in your private struggles, your shoulda, coulda, wouldas—those things are always gonna be there. I don't live in them, and I pull myself out of them, but there are a million of them. And, honestly, the more I learn about mental health and suicide, the more I'm like 'Why didn't I fucking know *that*?'" She put her hands on her head in utter disbelief. "How could I not know these things?"

So, I wondered, does part of this get worse? Because I see Solly as someone who is so good at being public about this—which is, of course, something I had to learn how to do, too, to be an advocate in this field. But when I was talking to Austin Moss about Solly, he pointed out that part of what makes professional athletes so extraordinary is their ability to do something amazing right in the face of the biggest adversity, something regular people can't do. And that is *not* the same as taking care of yourself.

"Right," Martha said, as Chris kept nodding. "Right."

I told them I wasn't criticizing. I just wanted to note that you can be a great public advocate and still be in private pain.

"That morning in Vietnam, Solly said to me, 'I think I have my grief under control,'" Martha recalled. "And I remember saying, 'Son, you don't get to control grief. That isn't what happens. You don't ever get to control it. All you can do is acknowledge it when it hits you.'"

What Martha said about extended grief is actually true of all mental illnesses and addictions. You don't ever get to completely control them. All you can do is acknowledge, diagnose and treat them, respect them, and get the people in your life to help you respect them.

All you can do is play defense.

Afterword

It has been a privilege and a powerful experience to bring these twelve *Profiles in Mental Health Courage* to life. But it has also been a uniquely emotional challenge.

After meeting with more than a hundred people to get recommendations for possible profile subjects and spread the word about the project, we did long initial interviews with over forty people, and then extensive follow-up interviews with more than twenty-five people—plus, in many cases, their family members, mental health providers, employers—before doing any writing.

We got to know a lot of people at an extremely personal level because, in many cases, they had never admitted—sometimes even to themselves—all the struggles they had endured to find and pay for care, maintain the support of their loved ones, hold on to their jobs and lives, and remain healthy. And, in fact, not all of them remained healthy during the process. As you can probably tell from some of the profiles, several of our subjects experienced major health setbacks during the time we worked with them to tell their stories, in many cases for more than a year. Some had breakthrough symptoms of mental illness or devastating lapses in their sobriety. We were with several people and their families through overdoses and hospitalizations. It was a constant reminder that while some people "come out" when they are at the peak of wellness, it takes a different kind of courage to be honest about your illness when you are sick, again, but still hopeful about the power of relationships and the value of care.

Still, it was hard to hear that someone we had gotten to know was ill, in danger, in some cases even missing for a short period. Sometimes people let us know in real time; in other situations, they waited until things had started to improve to let us know where they had been. The level of trust and openness was inspiring, and occasionally overwhelming. There were times when we knew things that family members, and even mental health providers, didn't know yet. In some cases, because we were also interviewing their doctors, we were the first to let them know about their patient's setbacks.

We did our best to be worthy of our subjects' trust—both in sharing what they told us and trying to create something useful and important, something with the power to transform the way people see and talk about mental health. We also kept our promise that they could withdraw from the project at any time, if they decided, for any reason, that they did not feel ready to be this open. In some cases, people exercised their option after meeting just once, especially when they realized we were serious about only profiling people who would let us use their real names: they just assumed, since so many people speak under pseudonym to avoid discrimination and stigma, that we would offer that option. But one of the most important reasons we wanted to do this book was to tell people's real stories, using their real names.

We also met several families we hoped to profile but their family member with mental illness was either not well enough to participate or, in some cases, to even acknowledge their illness. We felt we should try to focus on situations where the person with the illness was the center of our attention and could fully participate.

We had a handful of people withdraw after several interviews and in-depth sharing of their medical information—sometimes because they had relapsed, or because they worried that the book experience might trigger relapse.

And in at least one case, we had completed and fully fact-checked with multiple sources one of the longer chapters in the book, which was ready to go to the printer. After reading the finished version, which every profile subject was allowed to do before moving forward to publication, this prominent person (and a good friend of mine) decided, in consultation with their spouse and well-known employer, it was just the wrong time to be this open. I will never forget that moment with the profile subject we had spoken to so many times, who was choking back tears while breaking the news to us over Zoom from their car. We were crushed, but we completely understood.

There was, in fact, a moment in 2015 when I could have done the same thing with the completed manuscript of *A Common Struggle*—even though it was ready to be published and I had already been booked on *60 Minutes* to talk about it. Nobody but my wife, Amy, and my coauthor, Stephen, ever knew how close we came to calling it off.

I am forever glad, and proud, that we moved forward, just as I am honored that the people in this book stuck with it. And I will never forget the aching, moving discussions we had with them, when they shared things that, in many ways, they were astonished they had survived, as well as the long email exchanges ensuring the logistics and chronology of their stories were pinpoint accurate, the feelings surrounding their darkest experiences captured just right.

Stephen had done isolated interviews like this his entire career—including with me, and others in our field like Kay Redfield Jamison, PhD, the first legislative heroes of parity, senators Pete Domenici and Paul Wellstone, and the founders of NAMI. But he said he had never been involved this deeply with people and their families, especially with multiple stories at the same time, unrelated except that they were all part of *Profiles in Mental Health Courage*. And because we had asked people to request their medical records and contact their care providers, we weren't only relying on their memories alone. Just as I discovered so much about my illnesses from going through records with Stephen, in some cases we were able to help people connect the dots of their treatment and life experiences—and even alter the way they had been connecting them for themselves. As many of us with mental illnesses and addictions benefit from sharing our stories—in support groups, in therapy, with loved ones—there is also something transformative about the development of those stories into more reported narratives, like our own mental health biographies.

There were times working on this book when we truly could not believe what we were being told, either because it was so inspiring or so utterly heartbreaking. And I'm guessing there were times when our profile subjects were surprised by what I shared with them, because nothing in my journey through mental health and addiction care really seems like it is truly in the past. I don't presume it is behind me. Even though Amy and I have been together for well over a decade and have five children, I never, ever forget our first year, during which I was still drinking to excess and misusing prescription drugs. And yet we still fell in love. We celebrate my sobriety "birthday" of February 22, 2011, not as an increasingly distant memory but as a reminder that recovery is an active, daily process. And we are as careful about me staying on my meds—currently the mood stabilizer lamotrigine (Lamictal) and the antidepressant vortioxetine (Trintellix)—as we were the first time I took them in the context of a loving, supportive relationship.

I am supremely fortunate—for my life, for my family, and for my work. I am lucky to have been able to create a book like this, and I hope it helps encourage broader and more in-depth mental health family storytelling. I hope and pray that these profiles in courage can inspire, humble, and energize, and remind us that there is no health without mental health.

Acknowledgments

So many people, all over the country and all over the world of mental illness and addiction, helped us with *Profiles in Mental Health Courage*. Our record of calls and Zooms for the two years we worked on this is absolutely packed with fascinating and amazingly supportive people, so many of whom we can't name, as the whole goal of this process was to quietly spread the word to anyone we thought could help, but to keep their cooperation secret unless they were mentioned in the finished book. We did this because we didn't know which profile subjects would ultimately agree to let us publish the chapter we developed on them. We also didn't know how many chapters we would be able to have—each time a chapter grew longer and more in depth, it meant another chapter might not get into the finished book. But we are hoping this is just the beginning of creating and sharing these kinds of mental health narratives.

We first want to thank, beyond words, our final group of *Profiles in Mental Health Courage*: Philomena Kebec, Henry Platt, Gabrielle Anwar, Tonie Dreher, Justin Maffett, Ashley Dunlop, the family of Patrick's late cousin Harry McMurrey (Mark and Belton McMurrey), Bob Kazel, Naia Butler-Craig, Gene Barduson and Gretchen Ficek, Aidan Understein, and the family of the late Ella Thomas (Solomon, Martha, and Christopher Thomas). They have all selflessly allowed their personal stories to be shared, at a potentially high risk to them, to help our country overcome its denial of our mental epidemics. We have all been through a remarkable experience together with only one goal: to change the way people think and talk about mental health.

We also want to thank the people in the lives of these twelve who participated in the creation of these chapters and agreed to be identified. In order of their appearance in the book: Michael Botticelli, Mark Gardner, Hannah Lottenberg, Shareef Malnik, Dr. Charles Nemeroff, Dr. Elizabeth Ford, Dr. Arthur Evans, Rev. Al Sharpton, Drew Dunlop, Dr. David Markovitz, Garrett Laurie, Chad Metcalf, Jonathan Eig, Dr. Carl Wahlstrom, Nicole Lloyd-Ronning, Timna Zucker, Dr. Murray Zucker, Austin Moss, and many others who spoke to us for these chapters and chose not to be identified. Thanks also to those who devoted time, energy, and heart to the interview process, but whose chapters we were unable to include, and are acknowledged by initials until their stories can be shared: S.R., K.P., E.S., D.S., C. G-K., A.S., C.T., M.S., and A.K.

We are so grateful to the small team that worked on this book, in complete secrecy, for nearly two years: Diane Ayres, our amazing twenty-four-hour-a-day in-house editor (also an inspiring novelist and Stephen's wife); Meg Gladieux, our bright and multitasking assistant on the project (also a talented Penn-grad writer and editor); Kara Kukfa, Patrick's outstanding chief of staff, who keeps so many things in his life on course; David Black, our wise and fearless agent; and John Parsley, our enthusiastic and patient editor at Dutton (along with his wonderful staff).

Thanks also to those who we reached out to as "connectors" to help us find people who might be willing to, at least, do an introductory interview with us about the project, especially: Rebecca Bagley, Denise Bertin-Epp, Meiram Bendat, Courtenay Harris Bond, Mark Bradshaw, Tom Coderre, Brett Cooke, Jess Cordova, Phil D. M. de Picciotto, Dr. Steven Descoteaux, Hilary de Vries, Andy Dunn, Dr. Maurizio Fava, Seth Feuerstein, Dr. Richard Friedman, Dr. Andrew Gerber, Scott Gorman, Dr. Gary Gottlieb, Jesse Gould, Ryan Hampton, Dr.

Steve Hyman, Dr. Tom Insel, Dr. Nick Kadaras, Dr. Howard Koh, Madhuri Jha, Martin Luther King III, Dr. George Koob, Dr. John Krystal, Anna Lembke, David Lloyd, John MacPhee, Ron Manderscheid, Marjorie Morrison, Dr. Doug Nemecek, Dr. Maria Oquendo, Dr. Kathy Pike, Dr. Kelly Posner, Stephanie Prechter, Kathryn Ramstad, Dr. Scott Rauch, Linda Rosenberg, Dr. Ken Rosenberg, Todd Rudsenske, Dr. Estee Sharon, Dr. Jon Sherin, Andy Slavitt, Dr. Ron Smith, Senator Gordon Smith, David Smith, Andrew Solomon, Dr. Matt State, Dr. Paul Summergrad, Karen Swartz, Katherine Switz, Mike Thompson, Chris Thrasher, Troy Vincent, Jamie Vinck, Dr. Nora Volkow, Marty Walsh, and Dr. Glenda Wrenn.

For every one of these, there are many others who talked to us but chose not to be identified. The process of helping people come out with their true mental health narratives involves so many layers of confidences. We hope we have been successful in keeping all of them.

STEPHEN WOULD LIKE to personally thank Victoria Wyeth (who helped transcribe in the earliest days of the project); Jon Eig (who, besides introducing us to Bob Kazel, read other chapters for us); Geoffrey Little; my patient friends in Philly and the Southwest (especially the Last Supper Club, the Halfcourt Hoopsters, and the Santa Fe Six); my loving family; and the people whose mental health and addiction stories I've been privileged to cover over the years (* denotes a pseudonym): Marc Landis, Daniel Ferdock, Michelle Qurashi, Courtney O'Connor*; Jesse Foell; Michael Cowlin*, Kenny Gallery*, T. K. Fegley*, James O'Boyle; Eric Motis; Frankie Lymon, Elizabeth Waters Lymon; Gia Carangi, Elyssa Golden; Bill King; Anne Sexton; Kay Jamison; Steven*; Jennifer Freyd, Pam Freyd, Peter Freyd; Claire*, Lisa*, and other patients at the old Institute of Pennsylvania Hospital; Marie and Arthur

Noe; Michael*; Adrienne Bransky; the Gold Star widows of Killeen, Texas; Sigmund "Siggy" Miller; my uncle, Michael Fried; Dr. Aaron "Tim" Beck; and my friend, Major van Winkle, whose death by suicide I researched for the award-winning 2022 documentary *This Is Major.*

PATRICK WOULD LIKE to personally thank everyone at The Kennedy Forum and Alignment for Progress; my colleagues on the National Action Alliance for Suicide Prevention, especially NIMH director Dr. Josh Gordon (with whom I co-chaired the National Response to COVID-19); One Mind, especially my heroes Garen and Shari Staglin; the Kennedy-Satcher Center for Mental Health Equity, especially Dr. David Satcher, who has been so supportive in my post-Congressional life; and the CEO Alliance for Mental Health: Tom Chiodo, Shawn Coughlin, Lisa Dailey, Arthur Evans, Bob Gebbia, Daniel H. Gillison, Jr., Chuck Ingoglia, Rick Kellar, Andy Keller, PhD, Karen Larsen, Dr. Saul Levin, Danna Mauch, PhD, Angelo McClain, PhD, John MacPhee, Tyler Norris, Brandon Staglin, Schroeder Stribling, and Jan Wootten; as well as Chris Hirschy and Lorre Moylett, my scheduling and accounting assistants.

I'm also grateful to Allan Fox, Keith Lowey, and Peter O'Brien for their confidences and direction; my late cousin, Chris Lawford, who was so important in the early days of my sobriety and whose moving books and openness helped inspire our two books; and to John Z. and all of my anonymous fellows in recovery who help me trudge the road to happy destiny.

Finally, there are never enough words to properly thank my wife, Amy, and our five children: Harper, Owen, Nora, Nell, and Marshall. They are the reason I am able to live a healthy life and continue doing this work to help others. Their love and support anchor my stability and recovery every day.

AlignmentForProgress.org

Use this QR code or URL to access the Alignment for Progress site, where you'll find our National Strategy for Mental Health & Substance Use Disorders. The Strategy, the cornerstone of The Kennedy Forum's Alignment for Progress movement, is a first-of-its-kind, comprehensive set of recommendations for federal policymakers seeking to change the way mental health and substance use disorder care are provided, paid for, accessed, and delivered. Every part of the federal government has a role to play in our five areas of most crucial focus: prevention, early intervention and youth; parity, coverage, and equitable access; research and technology; emergency and crisis response; and workforce diversity.

About the Authors

Patrick J. Kennedy is a former member of the U.S. Congress, the nation's leading political voice on mental illness, addiction, and other brain diseases, and the *New York Times* bestselling coauthor of *A Common Struggle.* During his sixteen-year career representing Rhode Island, he fought a national battle to end medical and societal discrimination against mental illnesses, highlighted by his lead sponsorship of the Mental Health Parity and Addiction Equity Act of 2008—and his brave openness about his own health challenges. Soon after his father, Senator Edward "Ted" Kennedy, passed away, he left Congress to devote his career to advocacy for mental health. He has since founded The Kennedy Forum, which unites the community of mental health, and cofounded One Mind, which sponsors brain research and open science collaboration, as well as other nonprofit organizations addressing these issues. He lives in New Jersey with his wife, Amy, and their five children.

PatrickJKennedy.net

Stephen Fried is an award-winning journalist and *New York Times* bestselling author who teaches at Columbia University and the University of Pennsylvania. He is the author, most recently, of the historical biographies *Rush* and *Appetite for America,* and coauthor, with Congressman Patrick J. Kennedy, of *A Common Struggle;* his earlier books include *Thing of Beauty, Bitter Pills,* and *The New Rabbi.* A two-time winner of the National Magazine Award, Fried has written frequently for *Vanity Fair, GQ, The Washington Post Magazine, Glamour,* and *Philadelphia Magazine.* He lives in Philadelphia with his wife, author Diane Ayres.

StephenFried.com